Greening Health Care

Greening Health Care

How Hospitals Can Heal the Planet

KATHY GERWIG

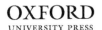

OXFORD
UNIVERSITY PRESS

Oxford University Press is a department of the University of
Oxford. It furthers the University's objective of excellence in research,
scholarship, and education by publishing worldwide.

Oxford   New York
Auckland   Cape Town   Dar es Salaam   Hong Kong   Karachi
Kuala Lumpur   Madrid   Melbourne   Mexico City   Nairobi
New Delhi   Shanghai   Taipei   Toronto

With offices in
Argentina   Austria   Brazil   Chile   Czech Republic   France   Greece
Guatemala   Hungary   Italy   Japan   Poland   Portugal   Singapore
South Korea   Switzerland   Thailand   Turkey   Ukraine   Vietnam

Oxford is a registered trademark of Oxford University Press
in the UK and certain other countries.

Published in the United States of America by
Oxford University Press
198 Madison Avenue, New York, NY 10016

Library of Congress Cataloging-in-Publication Data
Gerwig, Kathy, author.
Greening health care : how hospitals can heal the planet / Kathy Gerwig.
   p. ; cm.
Includes bibliographical references.
ISBN 978–0–19–938583–6 (alk. paper)
I. Title.
[DNLM: 1. Hospital Design and Construction—United States.   2. Conservation of Natural
Resources—United States.   3. Environmental Health—United States.   4. Maintenance and
Engineering, Hospital—United States. WX 140 AA1]
RA967
362.11068′2—dc 3
2014006487

This material is not intended to be, and should not be considered, a substitute for medical or other professional
advice. Treatment for the conditions described in this material is highly dependent on the individual
circumstances. And, while this material is designed to offer accurate information with respect to the subject
matter covered and to be current as of the time it was written, research and knowledge about medical and
health issues is constantly evolving and dose schedules for medications are being revised continually, with
new side effects recognized and accounted for regularly. Readers must therefore always check the product
information and clinical procedures with the most up-to-date published product information and data sheets
provided by the manufacturers and the most recent codes of conduct and safety regulation. The publisher
and the authors make no representations or warranties to readers, express or implied, as to the accuracy
or completeness of this material. Without limiting the foregoing, the publisher and the authors make no
representations or warranties as to the accuracy or efficacy of the drug dosages mentioned in the material. The
authors and the publisher do not accept, and expressly disclaim, any responsibility for any liability, loss or risk
that may be claimed or incurred as a consequence of the use and/or application of any of the contents of this
material.

9 8 7 6 5 4 3 2 1
Printed in the United States
on paper containing 30% post-consumer waste

CONTENTS

PREFACE VII

ACKNOWLEDGMENTS XI

ABOUT THE AUTHOR XIII

1. Launching a Green Revolution in Health Care 1

2. The Health Implications of Climate Change 25

3. The Business Case for Total Health 55

4. Food for Health 78

5. Managing and Minimizing Hospital Waste 106

6. Green Chemicals and the Detoxing of Health Care 132

7. Environmentally Preferable Purchasing: What We Buy Matters 164

8. Greening the Built Health Care Environment 191

9. Measuring and Reporting: Sustainability Gets Sophisticated 215

10. Community Benefit and the Determinants of Health 236

INDEX 253

The very nature of health care is changing. Health care reform, clinical innovations, electronic medical records, social connectivity, technological advances, baby boomers' expectations about quality of life, demands for price to align with value, and ways the environment contributes to disease are some of the factors behind the changes. These changes offer profound, new opportunities to address environmental issues across the health care sector and beyond.

In this changing landscape, what does environmentally sustainable health care look like? Let's take an imaginary visit to a hospital for a routine doctor visit. Approaching the medical facility, the first thing we notice is that the building is smaller than we expected. There is a convenient transit stop at the front entrance. And the parking lot pavement allows rainwater to filter through to be cleaned and returned to the aquifer. We notice that instead of lawns there are native plantings that minimize water and pesticide use.

There is a garden path that takes us by a stream that was brought back to life from where it was hidden in a concrete culvert decades ago. We enjoy the birds that have rediscovered this tranquil place. You notice a labyrinth and take a meditative respite.

Once inside, we are walking on nonvinyl, nonpolluting material on the carpets and floors, and we notice how much natural light floods into the lobby and hallways from specially designed window glass, shades, and blinds that allow sunlight in while minimizing afternoon heat. The walls are painted in soothing colors and patterns that mimic the adjoining landscape. The energy-efficient lighting fixtures glow with a pleasing hue. You see a plaque on the wall indicating that the building is carbon neutral.

In the bathroom, the toilets and sinks are water conserving, and the soap does not contain harmful antibacterial agents. The paper towels are made from 100 percent recycled, postconsumer waste, and the used towels go into a compost container. In the waiting room, the fabric on the chairs was selected to avoid harmful chemicals that can cause adverse health effects.

In the exam room, your temperature and blood pressure are taken with mercury-free devices. You notice the purple exam gloves used by the clinical staff. These are latex-safe for worker and patient safety, and they are environmentally preferable.

If you are here for a biopsy, your doctor will use a rigid endoscope (for minimally invasive surgery) which is steam sterilized to avoid the use of chemicals that are hazardous to the environment and to staff. Patients' X-rays are processed through a digital system that supports quality care by enhancing image analysis and transmission, and it is environmentally friendly because each machine eliminates the use of thousands of gallons of potable water annually as well as the chemicals and heavy metals needed for film processing.

As the housekeeping staff makes their routine rounds, we notice the absence of any chemical smells. This is because they use cleaning products that are free of harmful chemicals. And you see a cleaning system that supports zero waste through recycling, remanufacturing, and composting.

When we stop for lunch in the cafeteria, we have a selection of healthy options that are delicious, locally sourced, and sustainably produced, just like most of the patient meals. When we pass by the vending machine, we see a selection of healthy, nonsugary snacks and drinks.

This feels to us like a place of emotional and physical healing. We are better able to handle the medical issue that brought us here. We appreciate the sense of total health that surrounds us.

Everything we see on our trip exists somewhere in the US health care system today. In the future, we will see more of these features embedded in all care locations.

In my work as an environmental advocate in health care, I am often asked how people can best contribute to a healthy environment. There is much we can and should do to lessen our impact on the environment, such as reducing reliance on fossil fuel, preferring products that do not contain harmful chemicals, and being mindful about consumption and waste. I believe, however, that the best thing we can do for the environment is to reduce our own health risks, or if we are healthy to stay that way. The main causes of poor health in the United States are preventable: unhealthy eating, insufficient physical activity, tobacco use, and too much alcohol. One third of Americans are obese, and there is a tsunami of diabetics headed our way because millions of Americans are prediabetic today. Sedentary behavior increases the odds of cancer, stroke, depression,loss of bone density, and a host of other illnesses. The resulting response from the health care system to diagnose and treat these illnesses is environmentally intensive.

Health is determined by many social and economic factors, including education, community safety, employment, and culture. It is determined by physical environments that include food, media, and environmental quality. And it depends on access to quality clinical care and prevention.

As individuals, we can work to reduce our own health risks by eating healthy foods, moving more, and finding our joy. As members of our local and global communities, we can promote policies, programs, and innovations that make healthy behaviors the easier behaviors.

The greening of health care is a lesson of hope. And the future of health care holds a promise of planetary healing that extends far beyond the system of health care.

ACKNOWLEDGMENTS

Environmental stewardship is in the DNA of Kaiser Permanente. In the 1950s Henry Kaiser, the organization's founder, approved the installation of $5 million worth of pioneering air pollution control equipment at the Kaiser Steel Mill in Fontana, California. Founding physician Sidney Garfield promoted sustainable practices well before the first Earth Day. In the early 1970s, employees at the Kaiser Permanente Medical Center in Santa Clara, California, formed an Ecology Committee with an objective of teaching employees "ecological common sense." More recently, George Halvorson, KP's chairman and CEO from 2002 to 2013 regularly celebrated environmental stewardship accomplishments in his weekly letters to staff. Bernard J. Tyson, Kaiser Permanente's chairman and CEO as of 2013, and formerly our president and COO, ensured our operational commitment to sustainable energy and waste minimization by approving national policies in both areas. The organization's long-standing commitment to environmental sustainability is but one example of Kaiser Permanente's vision of what we call total health, a focus on the health of mind, body, and spirit that addresses the whole person, including the communities where they live, work, and play. I am privileged to be part of this organization.

This book would not have been possible without Jon Stewart, communications director at Kaiser Permanente until he retired in 2013. During the last few years of his career he committed his considerable talents as a writer and editor to this book. I am deeply grateful for Jon's approachable writing style, eloquence, and journalistic acumen. That this book has been completed is a reflection of his dedication and partnership.

Others from Kaiser Permanente who made significant contributions include Susannah Patton, who supported the overall project and helped author the chapters about food and waste, and Susan Saito, who helped write the chapter on green buildings.

Joe Bialowitz, a trusted colleague and respected expert, works with me at the national level to manage our overall environmental stewardship program. He contributed to several chapters, most notably the chapter on measurement.

I sincerely thank several external contributors, including Judith Nemes, Carrie Rich, and Seema Wadhwa. Their contributions are woven throughout the book.

Sustainability work at Kaiser Permanente is governed by the Environmental Stewardship Council. The Working Group of the Council is the home for our initiatives, and the members are an exceptionally gifted group of people who make their extraordinary achievements look easy. The Executive Committee of the Council provides wonderful inspiration and support while ensuring that the work is appropriately paced and focused. The chair of the Council, Raymond J. Baxter, took me and this work under his wing in 2007. I am profoundly grateful for his vision and mentorship.

It is my distinct honor to work with the amazing people of Health Care Without Harm. All proceeds from this book will be donated to that organization as they lead the global movement for environmentally responsible health care.

Kathy Gerwig is Kaiser Permanente's Environmental Stewardship Officer, responsible for organizing and managing a nationwide environmental initiative for the organization. Under her leadership, Kaiser Permanente has become widely recognized as an environmental leader in the health care sector. Kathy has testified twice before Congress on the need for federal chemical policy reform, and she has appeared at numerous hearings on environmental issues.

As Kaiser Permanente's vice president for Employee Safety, Health and Wellness, Kathy is also responsible for eliminating workplace injuries, promoting healthy lifestyle choices, and reducing health risks for the organization's 190,000 employees and physicians. She oversees the national departments of workplace safety; workforce wellness; integrated disability management; employee assistance programs; and environmental, health and safety.

Prior to joining Kaiser Permanente in 1993, Kathy was an environmental and economic development consultant to businesses and public agencies in the United States and Europe. Prior to consulting, she worked for nonprofit environmental organizations in California.

Kathy has a master's degree in business administration, with honors, from Pepperdine University and a bachelor's degree in geography and environmental studies from San Francisco State University. She is a certified professional healthcare risk manager, a certified professional environmental auditor, and a certified healthcare environmental manager.

Kathy is on the boards of several leading nongovernmental organizations focused on safety and environmental sustainability in health care.

Greening Health Care

Launching a Green Revolution in Health Care

Modern neonatal intensive care units (NICUs) are amazing environments. Nowhere else is one likely to witness, at a single glance, the utter fragility alongside the heroic miracle of human life. Tiny, preterm and critically ill infants—some so small their perfectly formed feet are no larger than a paper clip—lie enclosed in sterile plastic bubbles, surrounded by and physically connected to a stunning array of high-tech medical equipment that monitors and regulates their most basic biological functions. Highly specialized clinicians—neonatalogists, neonatal nurses, respiratory therapists, and others—move about the bassinets and bubbles with calm and purposeful professionalism, stopping here and there to bend over an infant with a smile and a coo, give a fingertip massage, and quietly confer with colleagues. Parents, exhausted from lack of sleep, keep a 24-hour-a-day vigil, unable to conceal that haunting mixture of fear, hope, and helplessness.

It was a visit to just such a unit, at Kaiser Permanente's San Francisco Medical Center, back in 2001 that left an indelible mark on my memory and has since informed my work as Kaiser Permanente's environmental stewardship leader and the way we deliver care to our 9 million members.

I was there with a small group of technical experts to follow up on suggestions from recently published reports that some of the medical equipment widely and routinely used in NICUs to provide infants with lifesaving blood, drugs, or nutrition might contain a chemical substance known as DEHP, or di(2-ethylhexyl) phthalate (pronounced "THA'late"). DEHP and other phthalates are used in polyvinyl chloride (PVC) plastic products to make them soft and flexible, and at the time PVC accounted for more than a quarter of all plastic used in durable and disposable medical products, including intravenous (IV) tubing, blood bags, gloves, and feeding tubes. As in other products, DEHP can leach out of flexible PVC equipment into the solution or medication it contains and subsequently into the patient.

In the late 1990s, several animal studies, including one by the US Centers for Disease Control and Prevention (CDC), had suggested that exposure to DEHP and other phthalates could be harmful to a developing fetus, especially to the reproductive system in males.[1] However, no studies had been done on human subjects, and because DEHP had been in use in a vast array of plastic products for four decades, the Food and Drug Administration (FDA) found no cause to test it when it began regulating medical devices in the mid-1970s.

Nonetheless, given the emerging data on the toxicity of DEHP in animals and other pollution concerns about PVC, in 1999, Kaiser Permanente joined a coalition known as Health Care Without Harm to petition the FDA to require manufacturers to at least label plastic products that could expose patients to DEHP. Without such identification, we had no way of knowing whether our PVC-based equipment might be harmful to patients, especially to susceptible newborns who often receive multiple and prolonged treatments with PVC-based medical devices. When that petition was rejected, the coalition published its own study, which laid out the known facts and urged health providers to seek out alternative medical devices known to be DEHP-free.[2]

With this as background, I decided that it was time to find out just how much equipment in our NICUs might be suspect. The group I assembled included experts in neonatal care, biomedical engineering, staff from our National Environmental, Health and Safety department, and Ted Schettler,

MD, the science director of the independent Science and Environmental Health Network, who had published some of the important research on PVC. At our San Francisco Medical Center, we were met by a wonderful neonatal nurse manager with more than a decade of experience in NICU care. We explained to her the facts as we knew them and that we wanted to inventory all PVC-based equipment in the unit to determine, if possible, which devices were likely to contain DEHP. The nurse was familiar with the fact that, during treatment, some plastic tubing lost pliability. But she was alarmed when she learned that it was because the potentially harmful chemical plasticizer was leaching into the solution used to treat the patient.

We catalogued item by item of invasive flexible plastic devices that, on later investigation, proved to contain as much as 80 percent by weight of DEHP: IV bags and tubing, umbilical artery catheters, blood bags and infusion tubing, enteral nutrition feeding bags, nasogastric tubes, peritoneal dialysis bags and tubes, and tubing used in cardiopulmonary bypass procedures, extracorporeal membrane oxygenation, and hemodialysis. Everywhere we turned in that sterile, caring, life-sustaining environment for sick infants, we found PVC-based devices that might contain DEHP, which was linked to reproductive and developmental damage to newborns, fetuses, and prepubertal children. The very equipment we were using to support life for these critically ill and preterm infants was capable of leaching a potentially toxic substance into their bodies that could result in reproductive abnormalities over a lifetime.

The sense of alarm soon turned to action. Following that visit and subsequent NICU equipment inventories, a technical committee of Kaiser Permanente neonatal experts directed staff to conduct a series of clinical trials to determine which products could be replaced with DEHP-free alternatives. Based on those evaluations, the committee moved quickly to switch to non-PVC/DEHP products for three of the most commonly used NICU devices such as catheters and feeding tubes. We also engaged with our main NICU equipment supplier to conduct an analysis of other products and non-DEHP alternatives.

Today, I am proud to say, the IV solution bags purchased by Kaiser Permanente are 100 percent PVC- and DEHP-free and our IV tubing is

DEHP-free. The product selection affects nearly 100 tons of medical supplies. As an added bonus, the safe alternative products are saving us close to $5 million a year.

In the meantime, the National Toxicology Program's Center for Evaluation of Risks to Human Reproduction has issued three reports on DEHP exposure to pregnant women, infants, and children, confirming that DEHP has been shown to be a reproductive and developmental toxicant in animal studies, and that those studies are relevant to humans. Other studies, from Harvard University School of Medicine and the University of Rochester, have gone further, confirming that infants subjected to intensive NICU care have increased levels of DEHP and other phthalates in their bodies, and that boys born to mothers exposed to high levels of DEHP display distinct differences in their reproductive organs.[3] Even the FDA, first in 2002 and again in 2007, has issued public health notifications outlining the risks of extended or frequent exposure to DEHP in high-risk patients and recommended that hospitals switch to a growing array of DEHP-free products whenever possible.[4]

After all these years, I still think often of that lovely and caring NICU nurse in San Francisco and her shock at learning that hidden in the life-sustaining equipment with which she lavished care on those tiny infants were chemicals that might, contrary to her every instinct, have contributed to serious health conditions for them years later. I suspect that the same emotions have played out among thousands of nurses and physicians in many hundreds of other hospitals over the years, as health care providers have begun to come to terms with the sometimes serious health consequences of an environment sickened by human-made poisons and neglect.

ENTER HEALTH CARE WITHOUT HARM

For me and for a handful of other health care professionals concerned for a healthy and sustainable environment as a necessary foundation for human health, that coming to terms began not long before my NICU visit. I tend to date the beginnings of the environmental stewardship movement in health care back to the mid-1990s, in my case, precisely to the day when I first met Gary Cohen of Health Care Without Harm in the lobby of the Royal Sonesta Hotel in Cambridge, Massachusetts. It was 1996, and I had flown in from Oakland, California, to attend an environmental conference sponsored by Tufts University. Kaiser Permanente's environmental stewardship strategies and goals were taking shape just as some important information was emerging that had direct relevance for health care, specifically involving the harmful health impacts of dioxin, mercury, and other chemicals. The conference promised to be a good opportunity for hearing the latest expert thinking on these and other issues I knew I would be dealing with, and for establishing a network of professionals with a shared commitment to environmental health.

Cohen, who was also attending the conference, had called me before that trip to introduce himself and tell me about plans for a new advocacy group called Health Care Without Harm that he was forming with Charlotte Brody, a registered nurse. I knew almost nothing about Cohen, except that he had a reputation as a committed activist with a focus on toxic chemicals. Health Care Without Harm, he explained, would be dedicated to cleaning up and limiting the use of toxic materials in the health care sector. This agenda seemed ambitious for someone who had no experience in health care. In fact, as I later learned, Cohen's formal training was in Eastern philosophy.

Nonetheless, a series of life-altering experiences, including Cohen's work on behalf of survivors of the 1984 Union Carbine pesticide factory explosion in Bhopal, India—which killed 3,000 people and sickened a half million more—had focused his activist's passions on the growing dangers of toxic chemicals. When the US Environmental Protection Agency (EPA) issued a series of alarming reports in the early to mid-1990s on the carcinogenic, reproductive, and immune system effects of dioxin, one of the most toxic human-made pollutants, Gary set his sights on the health care industry. Health care, after all, had been identified as the biggest emitter of dioxins into the atmosphere in the United States, due to the routine burning of thousands of tons of chlorine-based plastic medical waste and trash at an estimated 5,000 onsite or remote incinerators.

Brody, co-founder with Cohen at Health Care Without Harm, had come to focus on the same issue while serving as executive director of a Planned Parenthood affiliate in North Carolina. Her clinic routinely disposed of all manner of medical wastes, including PVC by incineration as a way of protecting patients and staff against the spread of AIDS. That seemed like the responsible and legal thing to do—at least until the EPA assessments on dioxin revealed that the main source of this toxin was PVC, which, when incinerated, creates dioxin pollution. "Most of us thought that the more we burned, the safer we were making our patients," she says. "We didn't know that every red bag (of medical waste) that we burned contributed to poisoning mothers' breast milk."[5]

PVC was and continues to be ubiquitous in health care in everything from plastic bags that contain intravenous solutions to exam gloves and even furniture and vinyl floors. It is plentiful, cheap, durable, and performs well. And as we have found over the past 15 years, shifting to less polluting alternatives has been possible for some but not all PVC-based products. Finding acceptable substitutes has been an ongoing struggle for many health care organizations.

PVC is but one of many disturbing examples of the paradox of health care's role in environmental pollution. In the course of providing health care to individuals, we are inadvertently using chemicals and materials that are hazardous to human health. We generate pollution and wastes that become environmental contributors to disease. Institutions dedicated to human health were among the primary culprits in poisoning the atmosphere with toxic emissions that, at even low levels, were contributing to human cancers and infertility. The fact that laws and regulations required incineration of many pathology and chemical wastes only made the irony more painful.

Health Care Without Harm was born out of that paradox. As Cohen puts it, "Health care is one of the only sectors of the entire economy that has an ethical framework as a centerpiece of its profession. Caregivers take an oath to 'first, do no harm.' But if you're running a hospital on energy that comes from a coal-fired plant, you are contributing to the asthma rate. If you have a McDonald's restaurant in the lobby of your hospital, you may be contributing to the rampant obesity rate and all the health and environmental problems associated with that. If I'm a hospital leader, I want to model for others to do the right thing from a disease prevention standpoint." [6]

With all this as background, I confess that I felt some trepidation prior to that initial 1996 meeting. As a representative of the nation's largest non-profit health care organization—and an industry known for caution and risk aversion in the face of major change—I did not know what to expect from this activist. Would I be viewed as the enemy, an unwitting agent of the chemical industry? Fortunately, any apprehensions I had dissolved when we met face to face.

Cohen and Brody's strategy was not to blame the health care industry for its ways. They were more interested in collaboration than confrontation, in working with partners rather than battling enemies. Cohen understood the issues surrounding harmful chemicals and products in the health care realm and in the interests of environmental and human health wanted to share what he knew. Brody approached the challenge from the same standpoint. Setting up the "good-guy activists against the evil, bad-guy hospitals," she says, "creates a dynamic where real change is hardly possible, and even if you do get some change, it doesn't create a trajectory of hope. Instead, if we create a dialogue among participants, all of whom have strengths and weaknesses, you can get much farther faster." [7]

I left that Cambridge meeting thinking I had established valuable contacts for the challenges I was facing, and I was determined to stay in touch.

Fifteen years later, when I reminded Cohen of that first meet and greet, he broke into a big smile. Recalling the days when Health Care Without Harm was more a vision than a reality, he said, "I remember going back to my colleagues and telling them I thought Kaiser Permanente was going to be a partner with us. It was like picking a lottery ticket from the ground and it turns out to be the winning number."

The payoff of our continuing relationship has been transformative for both of us. In many ways, our two organizations, along with several other mission-driven hospital systems that joined the movement early on, were embarking on a long and ongoing journey. Our journey would take those early concerns about environmental health and its links to human health from the fringes of the nation's health care industry to its mainstream.

Today, Health Care Without Harm includes nearly 500 hospitals, universities, health professional organizations, and environmental groups working in 52 countries. It has also created a separate nonprofit organization, Practice Greenhealth, which has become the nation's premiere membership organization for hundreds of large and small health care systems committed to environmental stewardship and sustainability (see Box 1.1). The movement Health Care Without Harm helped nurture has played a key role in the ongoing transformation of American health care from its long-standing sick-care orientation to a disease-prevention and well-care agenda. And in doing so, it has demonstrated both the potential and necessity of reaching beyond hospital walls to improve people's health and well-being wherever they live, work, or play: in neighborhoods and communities, office buildings and factories, schools and playgrounds. It has helped to turn visionary ideals about health, the economy, society, and environmental stewardship into practical, cost-effective, commonsense strategies for a healthier world.

FACING UP TO ENVIRONMENTAL HEALTH HAZARDS

But that is getting far ahead of the story. For the truth is, despite all that has been accomplished in the past 15 years—and the progress has been impressive by any measure—the health care sector is playing catch-up to an explosive growth in scientific evidence in recent years about the links between human and environmental health. As Susan Dentzer, then editor of the journal *Health Affairs*, noted in a 2011 issue on environmental health, we now know that "the environment plays a role in nearly 85 percent of all disease. Yet...what we know about that subject—as opposed to what we need to know or do to protect health—is at best an inch deep."[8]

What we know today about the scope of the problems is a mile wider than what we knew 15 years ago. Back then, Health Care Without Harm and its earliest partners, including the US Environmental Protection Agency (EPA), the American Nurses Association, and a number of private health care systems, were focused narrowly on the emerging evidence

Box 1.1   PRACTICE GREENHEALTH

Practice Greenhealth is a nonprofit membership organization founded on the principles of positive environmental stewardship and best practices in sustainability by organizations in the health care community. Practice Greenhealth grew out of the former EPA-funded Hospitals for a Healthy Environment (H2E) and, as a membership organization, carried on H2E's agenda for the virtual elimination of mercury, reduction of the health care sector's total waste volume, chemical waste minimization, and other educational and information-sharing activities. Its overriding goals include the following:

- Preventing, reducing, and generating less waste in the health care sector
- Achieving carbon neutrality in health care
- Reducing energy and water usage
- Encouraging responsible construction, renovation, and product purchasing
- Maintaining safe and respectful work environments
- Engaging communities on environmental sustainability in design, construction, and operations
- Increasing recycling programs
- Phasing out hazardous substances and toxic chemicals

Practice Greenhealth has more than 1,200 members, including hospitals and health systems, health care provider organizations, major health care product and service providers, plus architectural, engineering, and design firms, group purchasing organizations, and affiliated nonprofit organizations. It is the key sponsor of the Greening the Supply Chain Initiative, the Greening the Operating Room Initiative, and the Healthier Hospitals Initiative.

about the hazards of hospital-based PVC and dioxin pollution. They also took on mercury, a potent neurotoxin that can harm the brain, spinal cord, kidneys and liver, and was used widely in hospitals in virtually all thermometers, blood pressure instruments, and other medical devices. Today, thanks largely to Health Care Without Harm's early campaigns to inform health systems of the dangers of these chemicals and its work to find cost-effective alternatives, both hazards have been minimized, if not eliminated. Mercury thermometers and blood pressure devices are now practically obsolete in the United States, and only about 60 medical waste incinerators remain of the thousands that were spewing dioxin into the atmosphere 15 years ago.

Toxic Chemicals

Every year, the evidence linking costly and increasingly widespread chronic diseases like cancer, asthma, and Parkinson's disease to environmental factors grows stronger, including environmental exposure to tens of thousands of human-made chemicals. The chemical world into which most of us were born was a universe apart from the relatively benign chemical environment that greeted our parents' or grandparents' generations. And given the rate of production of new chemical substances, still untested for human health impacts, it is hard to imagine the chemical soup that awaits the next generation. In just the last 50 years, more than 80,000 synthetic chemicals have been invented and put to use in commercial applications. Due to weaknesses in the Toxic Substances Control Act (TSCA), we know practically nothing about the potential impacts on human health of the vast majority of these chemicals. Of the industrial chemicals that have been registered with the EPA since 1976, when the act was passed, approximately 62,000 were "grandfathered" into the inventory without any toxicity testing. Even now, new chemicals added to furniture, electronics, toys, cosmetics, household products—and medical products—can go to market with no proof that they are safe. Most hospital purchasing departments are in no better position to determine the health impacts of the billions of dollars' worth of products they purchase every year than the average consumer. And even after negative health impacts are documented, the TSCA makes it almost impossible for the EPA to ban products containing harmful chemicals.

Since 1999, the National Biomonitoring Program of the CDC has conducted periodic surveys of human exposure to 219 of the estimated 3,000 chemicals that are considered "high-production" chemicals, meaning they are produced in volumes exceeding a million pounds per year. The results are published in the *National Report on Human Exposure to Environmental Chemicals*. Over the years, measureable amounts of all tested chemicals have been detected in the bloodstreams and urine of virtually all Americans, including pregnant women.

GETTING PERSONAL

In 2005 I agreed, out of pure curiosity, to be tested for the presence of 27 common industrial chemicals in my body. It turned out I had measureable amounts of all of them, including some nasty ones. It also turned out, according to the physician administering the test, that my results were typical.

Was I at risk? Certainly. But how much risk and for what? No one knows. No one really understands, with much precision, the impact of this twenty-first century chemical tidal wave, except for the relatively few substances that have been directly linked to animal or human health effects. Since the early 1990s, much attention has focused on chemicals known or believed to contribute to disease and dysfunction in fetuses, infants, and children, all of whom are particularly sensitive to toxic substances due to their disproportionate exposure per pound of body weight. Scientists cite strong evidence that toxic chemicals are directly linked to the rising rates of chronic diseases in children, including asthma, birth defects, neurodevelopmental disorders (such as dyslexia, attention-deficit/hyperactivity disorder, and autism), leukemia, brain cancer, and testicular cancer.[9] One recent study, from the Mount Sinai School of Medicine, calculated that the costs of environmentally mediated diseases, including lead poisoning, prenatal methyl mercury exposure, childhood cancers, asthma, autism, and attention-deficit disorders, exceeded $76 billion in 2008, equal to 3.5 percent of total US health care costs.[10]

Contributions to Climate Change

But toxic substances are not the only poorly understood environmental health threat lurking in hospitals and homes. Even now, scientists alarmed by the potential health impacts of climate change are urging public and private health systems to prepare to deal with entirely new kinds of health issues. These include the possible resurgence of vector-borne communicable diseases like cholera, malaria, and typhoid in developed nations, where they have been virtually eradicated, but also rising rates of Western-style chronic diseases like asthma and other respiratory diseases in rapidly developing nations. The World Health Organization estimates that, due in part to climate change, dengue is now endemic in more than 100 countries, up from nine countries in 1970, and is now a threat to at least 40 percent of the world's population.[11] Climatologists predict dramatic changes in weather patterns and the frequency of floods and drought, which will result in unprecedented levels of human migration and the spread of once-isolated diseases and even new diseases. Whether or not one ascribes to the well-documented evidence on the human causes of climate change, its potential health impacts are beyond political dispute.

From my perspective, what has been particularly disturbing is the growing evidence over the last 10–15 years of the extent of the health care industry's own contributions to environmental pollution. For instance, we have learned that hospitals constitute the second most energy-intensive commercial buildings in the United States. Operating around the clock, they use more than 2.5 times the energy per square foot of other commercial buildings and make an equally outsized contribution to carbon dioxide emissions. One average-size US hospital produces approximately 18,000 tons of carbon dioxide annually.[12] Overall, US hospitals' energy demands account for about 8 percent of total US energy consumption, at a cost of more than $8.5 billion a year, and rising.[13] According to a 2009 study, the health care sector in the United States contributes 8 percent of the nation's total greenhouse gas emissions, which are at least in part responsible for rising levels of such chronic diseases as asthma and diseases of the lung and heart.[14]

Hospitals are also voracious consumers of water, which we only recently have come to regard as a precious and diminishing natural resource. Health care institutions are consistently among the top 10 water users in their communities, with typical use ranging from a low of 80 gallons per bed per day to as high as 350 gallons, or 250,000–700,000 gallons per bed annually.[15] And it does not stop with greenhouse gases and water. As noted, chemicals are particularly ubiquitous in hospitals, which are the nation's single largest users of chemical agents, present in the form of pesticides, cleaning agents, disinfectants, fragrance chemicals, building materials, and other products that, as they vaporize, contribute to indoor air pollution, which the EPA considers one of the most serious environmental risks to public health.

Then there is the simple matter of hospital waste—actually a very complicated matter when it comes to the disposal of biohazardous medical waste or the more common and voluminous nonmedical wastes. Hospitals generate some 7,000 tons of waste per day, or more than 2.3 million tons a year, which must be sorted into various categories for disposal at a cost estimated by the American Society for Healthcare Engineering at $10 to $15 billion a year.[16] The environmental consequences of this waste, when incinerated, include cancer and reproductive effects caused by the release of toxins, notably mercury and dioxins. Other waste incineration issues include greenhouse gases emissions, human health hazards, and explosions caused by the generation of methane gas from the decomposition of organic materials in landfills. Although many hospitals have long used onsite steam sterilizers to treat biohazardous waste and found them to be cost effective, some wastes are still required by law to be treated by high heat, and that usually means incineration. In 2010, Kaiser Permanente set an organization-wide goal to reuse, recycle, or compost at least 40 percent of our nonhazardous waste materials by 2015.

Within recent memory, many health care workers never thought twice about putting noninfectious wastes, such as paper and lunch containers, into the infectious waste stream, which ended up in incinerators or steam sterilizers. As much as 50 percent of supposedly hazardous wastes at many hospitals turned out to be completely benign. Once hospitals reviewed their waste volumes and costs, they realized that they could save significant money by segregating their nonhazardous from medical and hazardous wastes and by reprocessing or recycling much of it, including disposable, single-use medical devices. One large hospital system, the Hospital Corporation of America, eliminated 94 tons of waste in 2010 through reprocessing alone.[17] Yet despite these successes, better waste management continues to be a huge, low-hanging opportunity in the health care sector. This is the bad news.

FIRST STEPS ON THE JOURNEY TO SUSTAINABILITY

The good news is that the health care industry is rapidly waking up to its double-edged impacts on health and the environment and is making significant strides to become more environmentally responsible and sustainable. What's more, as Gary Cohen says, health care is one of the few industries that has the economic clout, the scientific expertise, the public credibility, and, perhaps most important, the motivations and mission to "do no harm" and to change practices that may cause harm, not only within its own sphere of operations but, through pressure on its supply chain, on a national, economy-wide scale. Generating about 17 percent (and growing by 2022 to 20 percent) of all US economic output, health care is capable of creating and leading a national, and even global, transformation that could incorporate environmental sustainability in every dimension of the sector's economic activity for the health and well-being of the world's people.[18] It is that realization that drives people like Cohen and Brody, that drives me, and that has inspired thousands of American hospitals and health care systems— and many more, worldwide—to take the first humble steps on an endless journey toward sustainable, environmentally responsible health care.

Looking back, it is hard to tell where the starting line was. As important as Health Care Without Harm has been to promoting a genuinely "green" health care movement, it did not create the movement. Prior to 1996, at least a handful of health care systems as well as freestanding hospitals had small programs in place to focus on creating healthier and safer patient and worker environments. Some systems, especially nonprofits, also had robust community benefit departments that were engaged with local communities to fund and promote health and environmental stewardship programs.

An important milestone for health care's approach to environmental and sustainability concerns occurred in October 1963, when the environmental writer and activist Rachel Carson, author of the then-controversial book *Silent Spring*, delivered the keynote address at a symposium of 1,500 Kaiser Permanente physicians and researchers. Her book, published in 1962, is today credited with having launched the modern environmental movement. But at the time—when backyard gardeners were blithely spraying DDT on their vegetables—Carson was under assault as a communist and a radical agitator by her critics, led by the American chemical and pesticide industries. As *Time* magazine condescendingly put it, her "mystical attachment to the balance of nature…and her emotional and inaccurate outburst in *Silent Spring*," would do more harm than good "by alarming the nontechnical public."[19]

If Carson didn't exactly alarm her physician audience that October, the petite, soft-spoken, 55-year old biologist certainly made them sit up and take notice. Her theme was "man against himself." In discussing the "extraordinary unity that prevails between [living] organisms and the environment," Carson pulled no punches in warning about how pesticides and "the poisonous garbage of the atomic age" were despoiling the environment and undermining its ability to sustain the near-miracle of life on earth.

"We behave," she said, "not like people guided by scientific knowledge, but more like the proverbial bad housekeeper who sweeps the dirt under the rug in the hope of getting it out of sight." Our actions, she warned, are "changing the nature of the complex ecological system, and changing it in ways that we usually do not foresee until it is too late."[20]

The speech, sadly, proved to be her last public address before she died of breast cancer in 1964. Her legacy of scientific insight and passionate concern for the interdependence of human and environmental health has marked her as one of the greatest thinkers and activists of the last half-century. And she left an indelible mark on the evolving values and ethos of Kaiser Permanente, where physicians and staff employed well after her address "remember" the occasion with pride.

As the nascent environmental movement grew in sophistication and numbers over the decade following Carson's death, hospital staffers who responded to the environmental concerns she raised began forming what today are known are "green teams" at some of our hospitals. They worked primarily on recycling and waste reduction. But the scope of their activities expanded significantly when a series of news reports in the mid-1980s began highlighting the direct connection between medical wastes and community health.

In a small town in upstate New York, local health authorities searching for the source of foul odors uncovered a warehouse, near a children's dance studio, that contained five tons of neglected hospital and medical debris, including surgically removed body parts and hypodermic needles. Within months, stunned firemen responding to a blaze in a Brooklyn warehouse reported finding 1,400 bags of bloody gauze pads, thousands of hypodermic needles, and pill bottles littering a space where vagrants had been sleeping. Then, in the most sensational event, stories appeared over a 2-year period about thousands of pill bottles, intravenous tubing, and hypodermic needles washing up on a 50-mile stretch of the New Jersey shore, causing the closure of some of the state's most popular beaches and resorts.[21] It became known as the "syringe tide." And although hospitals were not directly implicated as the source, the issue of proper disposal of medical waste was suddenly a national concern.

By the time I arrived at Kaiser Permanente's Northern California Region in 1993, the development of green teams was well under way throughout the region, thanks to the pioneering efforts of Tony deRiggi, a pediatrician in our Sacramento hospital. His expertise and willingness to share made him a favorite resource throughout the entire Kaiser Permanente system, and his grassroots passion inspired many in the organization to follow in his footsteps—a clear example of how a single champion for a cause can create a sustainable groundswell of activism. I got involved in creating a regional green team that brought together physicians, nurses, engineers, housekeeping staff, and others to discuss how we could influence operations beyond our own medical center to stimulate similar efforts across all 18 of our hospitals in the region.

Another important early player, based in San Francisco, just across the Bay from our own headquarters in Oakland, was Catholic Healthcare West, now known as Dignity Health. With facilities in California, Nevada, and Arizona, Dignity Health was, and remains, a West Coast health care heavyweight. It was engaged in a variety of greening efforts across many of its hospitals well before the creation of Health Care Without Harm in 1996, and it became one of Health Care Without Harm's first members. In the same year, the system took what was then seen as a bold step and released a public report endorsing the Ceres principles, a 10-point code of corporate environmental conduct that included an organizational mandate to report periodically on environmental management structures and activities.

Ceres, a nonprofit based in Boston, was launched by a group of corporate investors following the 1989 Exxon Valdez oil spill. The spill gave a black eye to much of corporate America and demonstrated the environmental—and public relations—costs of doing business as usual, with little heed for the environment and societal impacts. The Ceres Principles included commitments to the sustainable use of natural resources; reduction and safe disposal of waste materials; energy conservation and efficiency; reduction of environmentally harmful products and services; transparency on environmental impacts; and a mandate to reduce or eliminate "the release of any substances that may cause environmental damage to the air, water, or the earth or its inhabitants." What's more, it committed signatory companies to conduct annual audits of their progress and to publicly report their findings annually.

Over the years, Ceres has had a major impact on how many large and small corporations the world over conduct their operations with regard to the environment, human health, and social impacts. In 1997, it created the now independent Global Reporting Initiative, the de-facto international standard used by more than 11,000 companies for public reporting on their economic, environmental, and social performance.[22]

Dignity Health thus set a new standard by becoming the first health care organization to publish a public report on its environmental health activities. "We recognized we were blazing a new trail in health care with this public report, but we saw it as critical to our expression of our mission to promote health," recalls Sister Susan Vickers, vice president of Community Health at Dignity Health. "We were hoping we'd make it safe for other health care organizations to join us and see the whole industry change and move in this direction."[23]

As it turned out, no other hospital systems were ready to take the Ceres route. But in the years since, the Dignity Health annual environmental health report has served as a powerful model to inspire others to become ever more aggressive—and more transparent—about environmental stewardship, a role it continues to play. In 2001, Dignity Health was one of the first systems to switch their IV bags and tubing to a PVC-free product—a move that, due to long-term contracts and the complexities of converting equipment, took Kaiser Permanente another 10 years to accomplish. For me, Dignity Health has continued to serve as an inspiration and thought leader. Sister Susan and I often trade stories about the barriers to making changes, such as altering or discontinuing long-term supplier contracts, regulatory obstacles, and the frequent inability to identify alternative products that meet all of the quality, efficacy, and performance criteria required in health care.

There were many other early joiners of the health care environmental movement, with each organization pursuing a unique mix of sustainable activities. Fletcher Allen Health Care, the academic medical center for the University of Vermont, was an early champion of recycling and other environmental health programs. By 1998, the Legacy Good Samaritan Hospital in Portland, Oregon, completed construction of its Marshall Street Addition with virtually no PVC, no volatile organic compounds, and designation of an "urban wildlife habitat" on the grounds. And medical schools at Harvard and Emory and the School of Nursing at the University of Texas in Houston were among the early systems to adopt green building projects, including extensive use of recycled materials, sustainably harvested wood, rooftop gardens, and PVC-free piping.

Another critical development in the early years of the movement was the June 24, 1998, signing of a memorandum of understanding put together, with Health Care Without Harm's facilitation, by the American Hospital Association (AHA) and the EPA. The agreement, which set ambitious goals for hospital pollution prevention, became the foundation for a partnership of Health Care Without Harm, the EPA, the AHA, and the American Nurses Association, known as Hospitals for a Healthy Environment, or H2E. With funding from the EPA, it began hiring staff and reaching out to health care organizations with a focus on getting hospitals to commit to the goals of the agreement by becoming "Partners for Change." By 2006, H2E had 1,342 partners representing more than 1,604 of the nation's 5,000 hospitals. At that point, it was reorganized as a not-for-profit membership organization and, in 2008, renamed Practice Greenhealth. Today, Practice Greenhealth membership spans the health sector, including more than 1,200 hospitals, health care systems, providers, manufacturers, architectural, engineering and design firms, group purchasing organizations, and affiliated nonprofit organizations. I am proud to serve on its board of directors. In the green health care world, which now includes numerous coalitions and associations, it remains the go-to organization for educational materials, collaborations, technical support, and a vast and growing library of case studies from member organizations detailing their challenges and achievements in virtually every area of environmental stewardship in health care.

In recent years, the green health care movement has broadened its initial scope beyond toxics and waste reduction and disposal to include alternative energy technologies, green design and construction, sustainable food services and community farmers' markets, transportation, and promotion of a wide array of community-based environmental health initiatives. Likewise, the number of coalitions, partnerships, and support groups has grown apace. Most recently, in January 2012, a coalition of 13 major health systems, representing nearly 500 hospitals plus related organizations, formed the Healthier Hospitals Initiative to promote a coordinated, sector-wide agenda for designing, building, and operating hospitals in ways that improve patient outcomes, protect hospital staff, prevent illnesses, and create environmental benefits while also saving billions of dollars in costs. As of early 2014, 836 hospitals had signed on to endorse the Healthier Hospitals Initiative's agenda for specific improvements in six major challenge areas: engaged environmental leadership, healthier food, leaner energy, less waste, safer chemicals, and smarter product purchasing.[24]

Progress has been especially notable in the areas of hospital design, construction, and operations. The Center for Health Design has become an invaluable resource for research, advocacy, and technical assistance in evidence-based hospital design that maximizes both patient and environmental health and safety. The Center for Maximum Potential Building Systems partnered with Health Care Without Harm to produce the *Green Guide for Health Care*, a voluntary educational tool for sustainable design, construction, and hospital operations, including energy and water use, chemical use, infection control, and regulatory requirements. Launched in 2003, the *Green Guide for Health Care* standards were piloted in 275 hospital construction projects representing more than 40 million square feet of space. The *Green Guide for Health Care* staff has also collaborated with the US Green Building Council to develop a hospital-specific Leadership in Energy and Environmental Design (LEED) green building certification system—a particularly important development at a time when the health care sector is in the midst of major building boom. And the Healthy Building Network, founded in 2000 by leaders from various environmental health organizations, has led the way for the construction industry in transforming the market for building materials to promote healthy and environmentally responsible buildings in all sectors, including health care.

Every year, these organizations and others come together in a growing number of national and international conferences. The annual three-day CleanMed conference, organized by Health Care Without Harm and Practice Greenhealth, now attracts hundreds of participants from hospitals, hospital supply vendors, architecture and construction firms, and pharmaceutical companies, all eager to learn and benefit from the growing green health care movement.

Setting Benchmarks for a Greener Future

Despite the impressive progress since the mid- to late 1990s in the greening of health care, the fact remains that the industry as a whole was late in joining the environmental sustainability movement. A decade ago, when relatively few hospital systems had moved beyond the early stages of recycling and waste management, comprehensive environmental sustainability programs were already being integrated throughout the operations of many of the world's top-performing firms in industries ranging from energy production to high-technology, pharmaceuticals, mining, finance, and other sectors. Many of these early joiners of the sustainability movement had historically ranked high among the world's environmental bad guys. Driven by increased regulatory scrutiny and growing evidence that investments in greening could actually increase earnings per share, spur innovation, and reap major dividends in public relations, some of these industrial leaders have set a high bar on sustainability performance that most systems in the health care mainstream are still aspiring to reach.

A truly green health care industry may still be a distant goal, but at least today it really is a goal—embedded in more and more health systems' missions and strategic plans. Led by a green vanguard that includes many of the nation's top-performing health systems in quality of care and community engagement—systems like Advocate Healthcare, Bon Secours, Cleveland Clinic, Dignity Healthcare, Inova, Kaiser Permanente, Partners Healthcare—the health care sector today is approaching that delicate tipping point that can transform a trend into the kind of megatrend that redirects the mainstream and redefines the future. As Gary Cohen told health system leaders at a recent CleanMed conference, the movement's pioneers spent the first decade of the twenty-first century "just building the scaffolding" of a green health care system. The next decade, he forecast, will see "the movement become the mainstream by embedding sustainability into the DNA of twenty-first century health care."[25]

That same conference concluded with an awards ceremony that offered compelling evidence of the great distance health care has traveled toward a truly green and sustainable future. One hundred and forty-one health care systems, ranging from single hospitals to very large, multistate systems, were recognized for environmental excellence based on detailed reports on their waste and recycling data, environmentally preferable purchasing policies, climate change mitigation activities, toxic chemicals policies, food service and cafeteria practices, and a host of other sustainability criteria. All of that data were aggregated into Practice Greenhealth's highly detailed Sustainability Benchmark Report, providing a snapshot account of the breadth and depth of the sustainability agenda across the leading edge of the movement today.

The annual benchmark data show that in the areas of recycling, waste management, and energy efficiency programs, for instance, the leading systems in 2011 diverted some 65,000 tons of materials from landfills at a savings of more than $43 million—dollars that go directly to the bottom line of improved health care. Most of the 141 systems had a full-time, designated sustainability manager to coordinate green initiatives. Ninety-seven percent of the systems had eliminated mercury-containing thermometers; nearly as many had implemented policies against purchases of any mercury-containing devices; and more than half were virtually mercury-free. Similarly, substantial majorities had reduction programs in place for products containing DEHP and PVC. Nearly all the top award winners also had adopted environmentally preferable purchasing policies, which promote sustainability throughout the entire supply chain. In addition, large majorities had implemented healthy and/or organic and local food purchasing policies for patient meals and cafeterias.

Awards are nice, but far more important are the actual health benefits that our work in environmental stewardship has brought over the past 15 years for Kaiser Permanente's 9 million members and for the communities we serve. Those benefits derive mainly from the five areas we have prioritized for action:

- Responding to climate change and its multiple threats to human health
- Promoting sustainable farming and food choices to combat exposures to pesticides and other toxic chemicals

- Reducing, reusing, and recycling to eliminate waste and conserve scarce resources, both financial and environmental
- Finding alternatives to harmful industrial chemicals to enhance the safety and health of our patients, staff, and our communities
- Conserving water, the lifeblood of the planet

On each of these fronts, we and other leading health systems have adopted increasingly aggressive annual targets and innovative strategies that are demonstrably making for healthier communities, a healthier nation, and a healthier, greener, more sustainable planet. Hitting those targets, year after year, represents the kind of reward that is driving hundreds of others throughout the health care industry to look to the future of health care delivery through a green lens.

NOTES

1. Agency for Toxic Substances and Disease Registry, Toxicology Profile for Di(2-ethylhexyl) Phthalate (DEHP), CAS # 117-81-7 (September 2002), http://www.atsdr.cdc.gov/toxprofiles/tp.asp?id=684&tid=65.
2. Mark Rossi, "Neonatal Exposure to DEHP and Opportunities for Prevention" (Health Care Without Harm, 2000), http://infohouse.p2ric.org/ref/16/15702.pdf.
3. Jennifer Weuve et al., "Exposure to Phthalates in Neonatal Intensive Care Unit Infants," *Environmental Health Perspectives* 114, no. 9 (September 2006): 1424–1431; Ford Fox, "Phthalates Threat: Less Boy, More Girl," *US News and World Report*, November 17, 2009, http://health.usnews.com/health-news/blogs/on-men/2009/11/17/phthalates-threat-less-boy-more-girl.
4. US FDA Public Health Notification: PVC Devices Containing the Plasticizer DEHP, July 12, 2002, and April 24, 2009, http://www.fda.gov/MedicalDevices/Safety/AlertsandNotices/PublicHealthNotifications/ucm062182.htm.
5. Charlotte Brody, interviewed by Judith Nemes, 2011.
6. Gary Cohen, interviewed by Judith Nemes, 2011.
7. Brody, interviewed by Nemes.
8. Susan Dentzer, "Embarking on a New Course: Environmental Health Coverage," *Health Affairs* 30, no. 5 (May 2011): 810.
9. Phillip J. Landrigan and Lynn R. Gold, "Children's Vulnerability to Toxic Chemicals: A Challenge and Opportunity to Strengthen Health and Environmental Policy," *Health Affairs* 30, no. 5 (May 2011): 842–849.

10. Leonardo Trasande and Vinghua Liu, "Reducing the Staggering Costs of Environmental Disease in Children, Estimated at $76.6 Billion in 2008," *Health Affairs* 30, no. 5 (May 2011): 863–869.

11. WHO, "Dengue and Severe Drought," fact sheet, September 2013, http://www.who.int/mediacentre/factsheets/fs117/en/index.html.

12. Energy Information Administration (EIA), "2006 Commercial Buildings Energy Consumption Survey (CBECS): Consumption and Expenditures Tables" (Washington, DC: US Department of Energy, 2006), table C3A.

13. Healthier Hospitals Initiative, "Leaner Energy Challenge," fact sheet, http://healthierhospitals.org/sites/default/files/IMCE/public_files/press_kit_pdf/hhi_leaner_energy_fact_sheet.pdf.

14. "Estimate of the Carbon Footprint of the US Health Care Sector," *JAMA* 302, no. 18 (2009): 1970–1972.

15. Robin Guenther and Gail Vittori, *Sustainable Healthcare Architecture* (New York: John Wiley & Sons, 2008), 271–272.

16. "Sustainability Roadmap for Hospitals: A Guide to Achieving Your Sustainability Goals," http://www.sustainabilityroadmap.org/topics/waste.shtml.

17. Ingfei Chen, "In a World of Throwaways, Making a Dent in Medical Waste," *New York Times*, July 5, 2010, http://www.nytimes.com/2010/07/06/health/06waste.html?pagewanted=all&_r=0.

18. Centers for Medicare and Medicaid Services, "National Health Expenditure Data, Projections," http://www.cms.gov/Research-Statistics-Data-and-Systems/Statistics-Trends-and-Reports/NationalHealthExpendData/NationalHealthAccountsProjected.html.

19. "Pesticides: The Price for Progress," *Time*, September 28, 1962.

20. Rachel Carson, "The Pollution of Our Environment" (speech presented at Man Against Himself Symposium, San Francisco, October 18, 1963).

21. Associated Press, "Fifty Miles of Garbage Closes Jersey Beaches," *New York Times*, August 15, 1987.

22. Ben Tuxworth, "Global Reporting Initiative: A New Framework?" *The Guardian*, February 22, 2013, http://www.theguardian.com/sustainable-business/global-reporting-initiative-updates.

23. Sister Susan Vickers, vice president of Community Health at Dignity Health, interviewed by the author, 2011.

24. Available at http://healthierhospitals.org/.

25. Gary Cohen, speech at Clean Med 2012, Denver, Colorado, April 30, 2012.

2

The Health Implications of
Climate Change

"Unequivocal." That's the term used to describe the reality of global warming and climate change by the Intergovernmental Panel on Climate Change (IPCC), established by the World Meteorological Organization and the United Nations Environment Program as the preeminent scientific body on the subject.[1] In December 2013, I attended a roundtable in London convened by Prince Charles on the effects of climate change on the environment and public health. Experts discussed an October 2013 report by the IPCC aimed at policymakers, which stated that atmospheric concentrations of greenhouse gases (GHGs), including carbon dioxide, methane, and nitrous oxide, are rising fast, exceeding preindustrial levels by about 40 percent, 150 percent, and 20 percent, respectively.[2]

In its 2007 report, the IPCC stated that it is "very likely" that human activity—mainly the burning of fossil fuels that emit carbon dioxide and a variety of other greenhouse gases—has been the main culprit behind the recent and predicted pattern of rising temperatures, shrinking ice caps, and higher sea levels that is expected to extend far into the future. "Very likely" is explained as a probability between 90 and 95 percent.[3]

In the urgent need to understand and come to terms with climate change and the reality of superstorms and erratic climatic changes, US health care needs to be front and center. As recent disasters have demonstrated, many of the old ways of doing things, from building and running hospitals and clinics to caring for the sick and keeping the rest of us healthy may be largely unsustainable given the challenges of a warming world. The British medical journal *The Lancet* put the problem in simple but stark terms when it warned in 2009 that "climate change is potentially the biggest global health threat in the 21st century.... The impacts will be felt all around the world—and not just in some distant future but in our lifetimes and those of our children."[4]

THE EPIDEMIOLOGY OF CLIMATE CHANGE

Health care organizations can address both the symptoms and the causes of climate change, just as they do in dealing with diseases. But before making a diagnosis or prescribing a remedy, we need to be clear about the epidemiology of today's climate change. What are the main factors driving the phenomenon, and how do they differ from more routine changes?

The earth's climate has changed dramatically many times over the millennia. The sequence of those changes can be read in ice cores, tree rings, glacier lengths, ocean sediments, and pollen counts. However, those past changes, including ice ages and eras of global warming, can be explained by natural processes, such as volcanoes, spikes in solar energy, and higher or lower concentrations of atmospheric carbon dioxide (CO_2) and other GHGs from the decomposition of carbon-based matter. During warmer, interglacial periods, the higher concentration of GHGs acted like a blanket to slow down the loss of heat to space, thereby influencing the earth's temperature. As the earth evolved, this greenhouse effect was responsible for creating the atmospheric conditions that enabled plant and animal life to evolve (see Fig. 2.1).

Anthropogenic (human-origin) causes (see Table 2.1), especially the increased emissions of GHGs from the burning of fossil fuels and changes in land-use patterns that reduce forests and other carbon sinks, are the

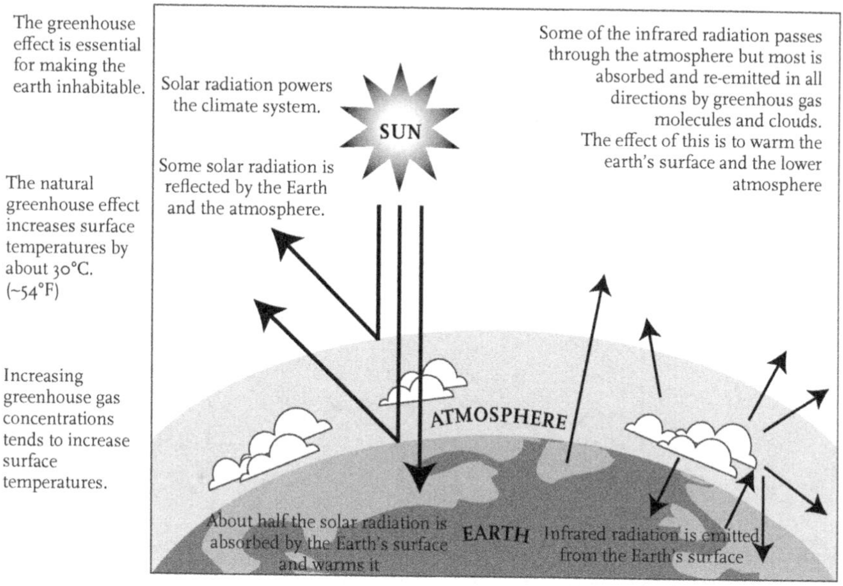

Figure 2.1

The greenhouse effect. The greenhouse effect is essential for making the earth inhabitable. The natural greenhouse effect increases surface temperatures by about 30°C. (~54°F) Increasing greenhouse gas concentrations tends to increase surface temperatures. (SOURCE: http://www.ipcc.ch/pdf/assessment-report/ar4/wg1/ar4-wg1-faqs.pdf)

TABLE 2.1 ANTHROPOGENIC SOURCES OF GREENHOUSE GASES

Greenhouse Gases	Sources in Human Activity
Carbon dioxide (CO_2)	Burning of fossil fuels, deforestation, cement manufacturing
Methane (CH_4)	Landfills, livestock, rice production, coal mining, natural gas operations, wastewater treatment, melting permafrost
Nitrous oxide (N_2O)	Fertilizer, planted nitrogen-fixers, combustion, medical gases
Ozone (at ground level)	Burning of fossil fuels and biomass
Industrial gases: Hydro fluorocarbons (HFCs), perfluorocarbons (PFCs), sulfur hexafloride (SF_6)	Human-made for industrial processes and medical anesthetic gases
Aerosols or fine particulate matter	Not gases. Burning and combustion of fossil fuels and biomass, among others
Water vapor	Power and industrial facilities, urban heat zones

SOURCE: Adapted from "Climate Change and the Role of Health Care Professionals," Practice Greenhealth Webinar, by Robert M. Gould, MD, April 14, 2011.

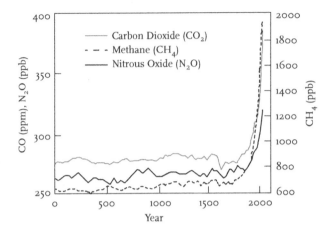

Figure 2.2
Rate of increase of three major greenhouse gases.
(SOURCE: http://www.epa.gov/climatechange/science/causes.html#ref1)

only way to account for the changes we see now. Human activities now account for the release of more than 30 billion tons of CO_2 into the atmosphere every year.[5] Figure 2.2 shows the increase in CO_2, methane, and nitrous oxide concentrations in the atmosphere over the last 2,000 years.

For the vast majority of climate scientists the most pressing question today is not whether or why the earth is heating and the seas are rising, but rather, What can we do about it?

"A MASSIVE THREAT TO GLOBAL HEALTH"

That question is finally beginning to be taken seriously by government agencies, major industries, and nongovernmental organizations (NGOs) all over the world. Its implications for key socioeconomic sectors such as health, agriculture, transportation, energy, water supply, healthy ecosystems, and civil society have been studied and debated endlessly by legions of eminent scientists and alarmed policymakers since publication of the IPCC's initial assessment report in 1990. Yet, to date, the growing awareness and acceptance of climate change has probably led to more sermonizing and hand-wringing than concrete action.

Anthony Costello, the lead author of the exhaustive 2009 *Lancet* study on climate change and its health consequences, proposed that health professionals should be spearheading three areas of action: First, they should be speaking out forcefully about "the threat to our children and grandchildren from greenhouse-gas emissions and deforestation"; second, they should be addressing and mitigating the "massive inequality in health systems throughout the world" in their ability to deal with climate change; and third, and most optimistically: "We must develop win–win situations whereby we mitigate and adapt to climate change and at the same time significantly improve human health and wellbeing."[6]

Dr. Dana Hanson, the incoming president of the World Medical Association, seconded those views in even stronger terms: "Climate change represents an inevitable, massive threat to global health that will likely eclipse the major known pandemics as the leading cause of death and disease in the 21st century. The health of the world population must be elevated in this discussion from an afterthought to a central theme around which decision-makers construct rational, well informed, action-orientated climate change strategies."[7]

Table 2.2 outlines a few of the major health-related impacts that tomorrow's health professionals will confront in a world that is just a few degrees warmer but a whole lot stormier than the world we know.

Climate change is expected to increase the prevalence of a wide range of health risks for hundreds of millions of individuals throughout the world, today and long into the future. Those risks are likely to be far greater for low-income populations in all countries, but especially in the developing countries in the tropics and subtropics. In these regions, rising temperatures, drought, and extreme weather events were already contributing to an estimated 150,000 excess deaths annually in 2000, almost 90 percent of them children, from rising rates of malaria, diarrhea, malnutrition, and other climate-sensitive diseases.[8]

Among the major climate-related health risks identified by the US Environmental Protection Agency (EPA) and other climate watchers are discussed in the following sections.[9]

TABLE 2.2 LIKELY HEALTH IMPACTS OF WEATHER EVENTS RELATED TO CLIMATE CHANGE

Weather Event	Health Effects	Populations Most Affected
Heat waves	Heat stress	Extremes of age, athletes, people with respiratory disease
Extreme weather events (rain, hurricane, tornado, flooding)	Injuries, drowning	Coastal, low-lying land dwellers, low socioeconomic status (SES)
Droughts, floods, increased mean temperature	Vector-, food-, and water-borne diseases	Multiple populations at risk
Sea-level rise	Injuries, drowning, water and soil salinization, ecosystem and economic disruption	Coastal, low SES
Drought, ecosystem migration	Food and water shortages, malnutrition	Low SES, elderly, children
Extreme weather events, drought	Mass population movement, international conflict	General population
Increases in ground-level ozone, airborne allergens, and other pollutants	Respiratory disease exacerbations (chronic obstructive pulmonary disease, asthma, allergic rhinitis, bronchitis)	Elderly, children, those with respiratory disease
Climate change generally; extreme events	Mental health	Young, displaced, agricultural sector, low SES

SOURCE: http://www.cdc.gov/climateandhealth/policy.htm

Excess Heat

The IPCC reported that the average temperature of the earth's surface has already risen by 0.8°C and is expected to increase 2°C–4°C by the end of the century. Even if only the minimum 2°C (3.6°F) warming takes place, it would be larger than any 100-year trend in the past 10,000 years.

The year 2012 was a record breaker for annual temperatures in the contiguous United States, according to data sets from the National Climatic Data

Center. As Figure 2.3 shows, 10 months in 2012 ended 12-consecutive-month periods that ranked as the warmest 12-month periods on record, with temperatures in excess of 3°F higher than the 20th-century average. The summers of 2011 and 2012 also ranked as the two warmest US summers on record, with one in three Americans (about 100 million people) experiencing 10 or more days of 100°F or higher temperatures in 2012.

Extreme Weather Events

Extreme weather events, such as floods, hurricanes, and droughts, are projected to increase as a result of global warming.[10] Average precipitation has already increased by 6.4 percent in the lower 48 states over the past century.[11] As with heat waves, the primary victims are children, the elderly, and people with chronic medical conditions such as asthma and cardiovascular

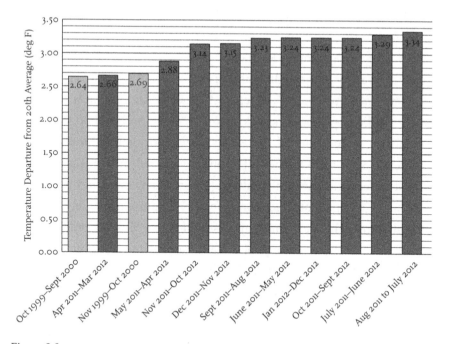

Figure 2.3
Warmest 12-month periods for contiguous United States: 1895–2012.
(SOURCE: National Oceanic and Atmospheric Administration's National Climatic Data Center, October 23, 2013. http://www.ncdc.noaa.gov/sotc/national/2012/13)

and respiratory diseases. The intensity of Atlantic hurricanes is expected to increase as the ocean warms. In many regions of the United States, heavy rainstorms that now occur at the rate of once every 20 years are expected to occur every 4–15 years, depending on location.[12] Heavy rains lead to flooding, which besides causing direct deaths and injuries can contribute to increased incidence of waterborne diseases due to pathogens such as *Crysptosporidium* and *Giardia*. The health consequences of increased downpours will be especially felt among the estimated 40 million people in the almost 800 US towns and cities whose sewer systems carry both storm water and sewage in the same pipes, resulting in raw sewage spills into lakes and waterways that supply drinking water.[13]

Not enough precipitation is also a problem. In California in 2014, rural communities are running out of water, and the drought is contributing to health effects from smog and particulate matter in the air. "We are on track for having the worst drought in 500 years," said B. Lynn Ingram, a professor of earth and planetary sciences at the University of California, Berkeley[14]

Besides threatening the health of individuals, major storms also represent a significant threat to many health facilities in low-lying coastal areas, as the city of New Orleans learned only too well during and after Hurricane Katrina in 2005, when historically high surging waters overwhelmed the city's levees, knocking out primary and backup power and forcing the evacuation of some two dozen hospitals.[15] More recently, Hurricane Sandy in October 2012 pushed a wind-driven tidal surge of almost 14 feet into lower Manhattan and forced an emergency evacuation of almost 1,000 patients, including many premature infants and critically ill adults, from the New York University Langone Hospital, and Bellevue Hospital—the city's flagship public health care facility. The unprecedented storm surges from the East River left the hospitals' basement, lower floors, and elevator shafts filled with 10 to 12 feet of water that knocked out the backup generators and fuel pumps, forcing them to scramble in the middle of a hurricane to get patients down darkened corridors and stairwells and into ambulances for transport to other hospitals.[16]

To prevent such disasters, hospitals in high-risk areas need to harden their infrastructure and do everything necessary so they can remain fully operational after a storm, says Spivey Lipsey, head of the New Orleans office of engineering firm Mazzetti Nash Lipsey Burch. "You have to make hospitals impact-resistant so they can withstand the force of hurricane winds, a deluge of rain, or a storm surge of twenty feet of water," he explains.[17] That entails placing the entire mission-critical infrastructure in a hospital above the height that a storm surge could reach—all electrical service, emergency power service and generators, emergency switching gear, chill water systems and pumping systems, onsite water storage, and domestic water and sewer capability (see Box 2.1).

Box 2.1 IN BOSTON, PARTNERS HEALTHCARE PREPARES FOR RISING SEAS AND STORM SURGES

After analyzing scientific data showing that the number of significant weather events and days over 90 degrees in temperature may triple during this century, the leadership of Partners HealthCare in Boston, which has an outstanding record in reducing energy consumption and greenhouse gas emissions, chose to act decisively. Special concern focused on the threat of floods from rising sea levels and future, severe storm surges.

"There's a lot of debate going on publicly about whether humans are contributing to climate change or if it even exists," says architect John Messervy, Partners HealthCare's director of facilities and capital planning. "Rather than wait for definitive proof, we're acting on the assumption that it's happening."

Partners HealthCare opened a 262,000-square foot, 132-bed rehabilitation hospital near Boston Harbor in the Charlestown neighborhood that was designed with the anticipation that the current sea level may rise 2 feet or more over time. Scientists predict storm surges inside Boston Harbor could lift that water level as high as 5 feet. With those predictions in mind, the ground beneath Spaulding Rehabilitation Hospital, which opened in April 2013, was raised with mounding before construction began. And to play it safe, the hospital's electrical systems, switchgear, and other operational functions were lifted up into the ninth floor instead of being placed in the basement, where they would typically be housed. Emergency generators, along with 5 days of oil to power them, are located up there, too.

Messervy says it cost Partners HealthCare a premium in construction costs of around 1 percent. "But it's a strategic approach to how to plan for climate change in the future. At the end of the day, we have to guarantee continued operation and clinical services in extreme weather events."

Perhaps the bigger challenge is retrofitting existing facilities to make them less vulnerable to expected rising sea levels. Massachusetts General Hospital, a Partners HealthCare facility located in Boston on the banks of the Charles River, has a dam separating it from the river. If that dam is ever breached, water will come rushing in, which worries Messervy and his colleagues. "We're developing a strategy that plays out over many years because we won't necessarily be able to fix it right away," he concedes. "We're rebuilding our campus all the time and we've factored in climate change concerns in our overall strategy."[18]

Air Pollution

Despite several decades of improved air quality in the United States, four of ten Americans, including those in nearly every major city, still live in areas where air pollution levels endanger lives, according to the American Lung Association's 2013 State of the Air report.[19] In California, air pollutants are estimated to cause 8,800 deaths and more than $1 billion in health care costs every year.[20] Climate scientists predict that things will only get worse as warmer temperatures increase ground-level ozone, which can damage lung tissue and inflame airways, aggravating asthma and other chronic lung diseases and contributing to premature death. Even if levels of air pollutants—mainly ozone and fine particulate matter from power plants, gasoline and diesel engines, and increased numbers of wildfires—remained at today's levels until 2050, warming from climate change alone could increase the number of Red Ozone Alert Days by 68 percent in the 50 largest US cities.[21]

Food-, Water-, and Insect-Borne Diseases

A warmer, wetter climate is expected to enhance the spread of pathogens transmitted through food, water, insects, and animals, resulting in increased incidence of gastroenteritis and food poisoning from salmonella. Also, the geographic range of ticks and mosquitoes that carry Lyme disease, West Nile virus, and dengue fever is expanding as a result of rising temperatures. West Nile virus, for instance, which is contracted from infected mosquitoes, initially appeared in the United States in 1999 when the virus, originally limited to Uganda, appeared in New York City. By 2012, it had spread to more than a dozen states, infecting more than 4,500 people and causing 183 deaths within 9 months and requiring officials in Dallas to blanket the city with a mosquito pesticide.[22] The incidence of dengue has increased 30-fold over the last 50 years. Up to 50 to 100 million infections are now estimated to occur annually in more than 100 endemic countries, putting almost half of the world's population at risk.

THE POLICY RESPONSE TO CLIMATE CHANGE

The World Health Organization (WHO) has observed that the predicted health hazards of climate change "are diverse, global, and probably irreversible over human time scales."[23]

But although the United Nations, WHO, the IPCC, and an alphabet soup of governmental and nongovernmental health agencies and commissions are actively engaged in scientific research and advocacy campaigns on the health impacts of climate change, WHO nonetheless concludes that "a comprehensive strategy to support a public health response is conspicuously lacking."

In the United States, the Centers for Disease Control and Prevention (CDC), the Federal Emergency Management Agency (FEMA), and the

US EPA, among others, have assumed the principal responsibility for planning and supporting a variety of climate-related adaptation and mitigation strategies, especially those related to illnesses associated with extreme heat. These strategies include federal efforts to track changes in environmental conditions and related disease risk, improving capacity for modeling and forecasting climate change and health effects, identifying the populations and locations most vulnerable to climate-related illnesses, convening public–private partnerships to address climate-related health issues, and developing and implementing preparedness and disaster response plans. Yet to date, the CDC's own climate change policy acknowledges that "the public health effects of climate change remain largely unaddressed."[24] There is no coordinated, long-range action plan to address existing or anticipated public health needs. As George Luber, associate director for climate change at the CDC, stated in 2012, "We've just started to pry open the door to get public health a seat at the table."[25]

The situation is not much better at most state or local levels. A 2013 study by the nonprofit Trust for America's Health found that only 15 states had published climate change adaptation plans that include understanding and planning for the changing risk for emerging and re-emerging infectious diseases due to changing weather patterns.[26]

Preparedness for climate change is not much better in the one private sector industry that one would expect to be a leader in risk management and disclosure—the insurance industry, including major property and casualty insurers, life insurers, and health insurers. A 2013 report by Ceres examined climate change activities and disclosure statements by 184 insurers in California, Washington, and New York—all states that require insurers to disclose their climate risk assessments and activities. These firms represent a significant majority of the US insurance market. Yet only 23 of the 189 insurers reported having a comprehensive strategy to deal with climate change, and most of those were foreign owned. What's more, "many (insurance) companies view climate change as an environmental issue immaterial to their business," according to the report.[27] One of the largest health insurers in the study even asserted that public disclosures were unnecessary "due to the lack of conclusive data linking immediate health effects directly (or indirectly) to climate change." Only one health organization, Kaiser Permanente, which integrates health benefits coverage with health care delivery, was the only company with an insurance component that was included among the top 10 companies cited for having "a strong climate position." This is a fact that none of us at Kaiser Permanente finds much satisfaction in.

HEALTH CARE CAN'T WAIT

While political battles over the reality of climate change and the related ideological disputes over energy policy have no doubt contributed to the failure to mount a robust national or international response, dozens of individual health care systems in the United States and elsewhere—especially those systems that deliver care—are stepping up to the challenge. For these systems, climate change, to a great extent, is not so much a new challenge as another, more focused lens for understanding and responding to many of the same environmental health threats that motivated them to become involved in the health care sustainability movement in the first place.

Targeting Greenhouse Gases

Among the top priorities for hospitals and health care systems is the pervasive challenge of limiting the health sector's own role in driving climate change, especially the emissions of greenhouse gases. As noted previously, the health sector is a major energy hog and a leading contributor of the greenhouse gas emissions that are the primary culprits behind global warming and climate change. According to the US EPA, America's more than 3,000 large hospitals consumed 5.5 percent of the total delivered energy used by commercial buildings in the United States in 2007, though they accounted for less than 2 percent of all commercial floor space.[28] In 2009, University of Chicago researchers, in a first-of-its-kind calculation of US health care's carbon footprint, reported that the health care sector accounted for nearly a tenth of the country's total carbon dioxide emissions, primarily from energy use by hospitals.[29] The US EPA estimates that 30 percent of health care's energy use could be reduced—a fact borne out by European and Canadian hospitals that consume roughly half the energy of their US counterparts without sacrificing quality of care.[30] Devising and adopting a broad range of efficiency strategies to curtail energy use or switching to non-carbon-based fuels in order to limit GHG emissions is thus a top priority for the health care sector.

The first challenge for hospitals and health systems is to figure out how much GHGs they are producing and where it is coming from—something that until just a few years ago virtually no one in health care knew or cared about. Today, there are numerous tools available for measuring GHG emissions, ranging from calculators designed for general industry to site-specific hospital audits performed by consultants. On its website, Practice Greenhealth lists several of the most common tools used by its members, including the US EPA's EnergyStar Portfolio Manager; the GHG Reporting Protocol (a partnership between the World Resources Institute and the World Business Council for Sustainable Development); the Climate Registry Information System, developed by The Climate Registry, a nonprofit consortium of North American states, provinces, and territories; and the Greenhouse Gas Management Institute, an international nonprofit training and education organization. Kaiser Permanente makes use of several of these tools.

IMPLEMENTING A SUSTAINABLE ENERGY POLICY AT KAISER PERMANENTE

Kaiser Permanente was proud to become the first health care organization in the nation to begin monitoring and publicly reporting our GHG emissions, beginning in 2005 in our California regions. Over the next few years we expanded the data collection and reporting to the District of Columbia and the eight states where we have operations. By 2010, we were able to collect data on all our Scope 1 direct emissions (from use of natural gas, medical gases, diesel, refrigerants, and fuel for more than 1,300 fleet vehicles), plus Scope 2 indirect emissions from purchased electricity. That annual effort involved getting data from 859 sites, including hospitals, medical clinics, office buildings, data centers, and other facilities. Our 2010 total emissions were 859,000 metric tons of CO_2 equivalent (a measure of GHG's greenhouse warming potential).

In late 2011 we developed, and senior leadership adopted, a Sustainable Energy Policy that calls for a reduction in our absolute GHG emissions of 30 percent from our 2008 baseline by 2020. This absolute target means that even though we project to increase our square footage, the energy we will use in the future will be cleaner and emit 30 percent less GHGs (see Fig. 2.4).

How will we achieve this ambitious goal? Our policy calls for four main strategies:

- Design energy efficiency into new buildings.
- Increase energy conservation in existing buildings.
- Develop onsite renewable and sustainable energy sources, including solar, wind, geothermal, and fuel cells.
- Purchase offsite renewable energy as well as renewable energy credits (RECs).

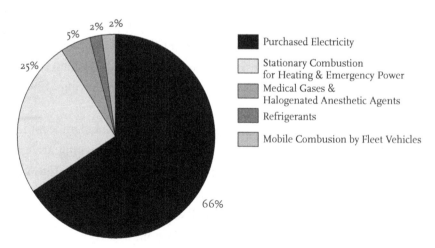

Metric tons CO_2 emissions = 796,106
(includes renewable energy certificates and carbon offsets)

Figure 2.4
Greenhouse gas emissions by Kaiser Permanente in 2012.
(SOURCE: Greenhouse gas emissions inventory prepared by Kaiser Permanente and assured by an independent third party.)

Additional priorities aimed specifically at reduction of GHG emissions include improving the efficiency of our more than 1,300 fleet vehicles and providing charging stations for electric vehicles. We are also focusing on ways to recycle emissions of waste anesthetic gases (WAGs), including nitrous oxide ("laughing gas") and various hydroflourocarbons, which have extremely high global warming potential and are typically vented directly into the atmosphere. The global warming potential of these halogenated anesthetics is up to 2,000 times greater than carbon dioxide (CO_2).[31]

According to Joe Bialowitz, principal environmental stewardship consultant at Kaiser Permanente, as much as half of the targeted 30 percent reduction in GHGs could come from relatively simple energy efficiency initiatives already in place or planned at existing facilities, including newer, more efficient technologies like the latest heating, ventilation, and air conditioning (HVAC) systems, window film installations, and energy-efficient lighting. "We knew that if we simply started ordering 25-watt fluorescent bulbs and installing them in place of the usual 32-watt bulbs," said Bialowitz, "this would eventually reduce the electricity use and associated emissions, and would be significant because lighting accounts for about 17 percent of overall energy use at health care facilities." We also switched out halogen bulbs for LED bulbs in surgical lights for a 33 percent energy savings and cut heat emissions by 34 percent, saving $109,000 annually.

Not all the upgrades are so simple, and some represent significant upfront costs. In all, the efficiency improvements we are making are estimated to cost as much as $16 million annually through 2020. That sum will be partially financed by working with energy service companies (known as ESCOs) that design and install energy efficiency solutions and are paid from guaranteed savings in the customer's energy costs over a number of years.

Other ways to get around or reduce the direct financing barrier include energy audits, rebates, and other assistance for efficiency upgrades offered by local utilities, and tax credits, incentives, and rebates available from federal, state, and local governments.

Moving to Renewable Energy Sources

Since the Industrial Revolution, increased efficiency has not resulted in reduced consumption, the so-called Jevons paradox. Therefore, the most important component of a GHG reduction strategy is sourcing renewable power. Bialowitz notes that we are also making major gains against GHG emissions from renewable and sustainable energy sources, both onsite and offsite, including solar, wind, fuel cells, and renewable energy credits. Between 2010 and 2012, we added 11 megawatts of solar installations at 12 of our facilities in California, enough to provide electricity for about 1,000 homes or to avoid approximately 7,300 metric tons of GHG emissions annually. In 2011, we also added a total of 4 megawatts of onsite solid oxide fuel cells at seven facilities, which we estimated would reduce each building's fossil-fuel electric demand by a third. Although fuel cells run on natural gas, these solid oxide fuel cells have the potential to run on 100 percent directed biogas, a non-fossil methane derived from landfills or manure.

Finally, we are supporting new, clean wind power by purchasing Green-e Energy renewable energy certificates (RECs). RECs are a way of guaranteeing that a share of the energy purchased for electricity consumption is added to the utility's power grid from a renewable energy generator, such as a wind farm, thereby reducing GHG emissions and providing an incentive for renewable energy generators. The RECs avoided approximately 12,700 metric tons of GHG emissions in 2011. Building on that effort, we are purchasing RECs from wind-generated power sources equivalent to 100 percent of our annual electricity use in 2012 and 2013 in our Maryland and Washington, DC facilities, thus avoiding another 54,000 metric tons of emissions each year.

"We're not putting all of our eggs in one basket," says H. Ramé Hemstreet, Kaiser Permanente's vice president and sustainable resources officer. "That's important because we don't know how it's all going to play out. At this point, we don't know which technologies or strategies will win out in the end, so it's important to spread the risk. In the meantime, we're supporting new technologies and helping them to succeed. It's good to be a part of that."

Designing Healthier Hospitals

As for new construction, the potential for major gains in GHG emission reductions is already evident at several Kaiser Permanente hospitals that have recently opened or are near completion. Our new 122-bed Westside Medical Center in Hillsboro, Oregon, near Portland, which opened in August 2013, is our first LEED Gold-certified hospital, and the first in the Portland area. We purchased 100 percent renewable energy from Portland General Electric throughout construction, and we have continued to rely on green power for a portion of the facility's power since its opening. The facility features high-efficiency heating/cooling equipment and pumps, co-generation heating systems (which uses steam left over from electricity generation and surgical sterilization to produce heat), as well as solar panels on the parking garage. The entire building is designed to optimize the use of natural light to reduce electricity use and enhance patient comfort and care. And to conserve water, all rainwater is collected in underground tanks and pumped via solar-generated power to irrigate the landscaping.

Dan Green, head of the hospital's green power initiatives, says that the potential contribution that Westside Medical Center will make in reducing greenhouse gases is projected to be just over 11,900 metric tons per year. "According to U.S. EPA data," he adds, "that's the equivalent of taking 1,000 cars off the road for a full year, every year, permanently."[32]

A big part of that emissions reduction will come from the hospital's eight-story parking garage, which is required by local building codes to provide all-night lighting. Thanks to photoelectric and motion sensors throughout the structure, all lights will be dimmed or turned on and off according to demand. Glossy white ceiling paint that reflects light will reduce the need for fixtures by 50 percent while maintaining brightness. As a result, the building will use just 25 percent of the power permitted by the building code. Jessica Rose, a business sector manager at Energy Trust of Oregon, says she expects the garage lighting alone to avoid using 300,000 annual kilowatt-hours, which is enough to power 27 Oregon homes.[33]

Zeroing In on Carbon Neutrality

In early 2011, faced with the emerging need for smaller hospitals to serve members in outlying suburban communities rather than the large medical centers in central cities, we launched a design competition for a small, green, patient- and family-friendly hospital that uses the best new patient care technology while operating with virtually zero environmental impact from energy use. More than 300 teams from 32 countries submitted design concepts. Following an 11-month evaluation by a jury of experts in architectural design and engineering, hospital administration, and clinical patient care, a partnership consisting of Aditazz and Mazxetti Nash Lipsey Burch, with Perkins+Will, was named the winner. The winning concept not only transforms the process of receiving and giving care by reconfiguring the relationships among patients, physicians, technology, and nature but also actually goes beyond our carbon neutrality requirement to include restoring degraded ecosystems and biodiversity while improving conditions for the health of the entire community. The so-called regenerative systems design significantly reduces demand for all resources, minimizes the generation of waste, and emits *no* greenhouse gases to the atmosphere and *no* harmful contaminants to the water cycle. These concepts will influence designs for our future small hospitals, beginning with one in Lancaster, California.

Advocating for Policy Change

A good example of advocacy in favor of reduced greenhouse gas emissions was Proposition 23 on the California ballot in 2010. Promoted mainly by out-of-state oil interests, it would have frozen implementation of the state's unique 2006 legislation on global warming, which requires greenhouse gas emissions in the state to be cut to 1990 levels by 2020 in a gradual process beginning in 2012. Physicians and public health experts spoke out about the health effects of climate change and air pollution. In the end, thanks to a coalition of health care advocates, the measure was soundly defeated at the polls.

Dignity Health's Energy Commitment

Kaiser Permanente certainly is not the only system making significant headway in moving beyond fossil fuels. Our San Francisco–based neighbor, Dignity Health, announced a commitment in 2011 to reduce its systemwide energy consumption by 20 percent and its overall GHG emissions from each hospital by 40 percent by 2020, partly by installing renewable energy sources for at least 35 percent of its systemwide energy use. Dignity Health, which has been a step ahead of most health systems in environmental sustainability, plans to achieve these reductions through a combination of energy efficiency upgrades and renewable sources, including photovoltaic, solar hot water, cogeneration, and fuel cell technology.

Gundersen Lutheran's Ambitious Quest for Energy Independence

And then there is a wildly innovative health system in La Crosse, Wisconsin. Gundersen Lutheran Health System, which serves patients in western Wisconsin, northeastern Iowa, and southeast Minnesota, is led by CEO Jeff Thompson, MD, winner of the 2013 White House Champion of Change award for climate and health. Gundersen Lutheran will radically change the way it powers its operations, having set a goal to be carbon neutral by 2014. To reach that finish line, in May 2008 the hospital system established a for-profit subsidiary called GL Envision LLC to manage the revamping of its entire energy strategy. In the first 18 months of the program, Envision was able to shave off 20 percent of Gunderson's energy consumption per square foot through a variety of strategies, according to Jeff Rich, Envision's executive director. The three key areas Envision focused on were energy, waste management and recycling, and sustainable design.

"It all started with an audit in 2008 to find cost savings, and we found we had a lot of opportunity to save money on energy with easy cost-saving fixes through conservation, getting rid of duplicate capacity, lighting retrofits and other efforts," recalls Rich.[34]

Initially, they focused on a retrocommissioning audit—a systematic, detailed study of building operations that identifies problems and potential, low-cost improvements, especially for energy-using equipment. Initial upgrades focused on systems that had the worst energy

intensity and included such things as adjusting boiler controls, installing energy-efficient lighting, and reprogramming the cooling system
to reduce consumption. These early efforts, says Rich, resulted in
$1 million in annual savings by the end of 2009. Having harvested the
low-hanging opportunities, they turned their sites to bigger challenges.

"We asked ourselves what would really make a difference here if we
really cared about the environment and the health of our community?"
says Rich. "Fossil fuel emissions cause cancer and are responsible for other
illnesses. You might debate climate change, but these health connections
aren't debated. It's known that emissions from coal fire (which is a dominant energy source in the upper Midwest) are linked to liver and kidney
disease and reproductive problems, too. Our mission is to prevent and
cure diseases, but we've been contributing to those problems in a disproportionate way. Our goal of moving away from fossil fuels ties into our
core mission of keeping people healthy."

Initially, Rich and his colleagues focused on deriving all of their future
energy needs from wind power projects, but that concept quickly morphed
into a mix of imaginative programs.

On the wind front, Envision created a joint venture with a for-profit
partner, and together they erected two large wind turbines in Lewiston,
Wisconsin, that generate close to 5 megawatts of power a year. Another
partnership, with Organic Valley, the nation's largest cooperative of
organic farmers, financed construction of two wind turbines at the
nearby Cashton Greens Wind Farm, which went live in 2012, generating close to 5 megawatts of energy for Cashton's power grid. The two
combined wind projects are expected to represent about 12 percent of
Gundersen's energy needs.[35]

Other innovative efforts will give the system even bigger bang for
their investment bucks. A massive boiler, fueled by woody biomass, will
replace natural gas boilers at Gundersen's La Crosse Medical Center
campus, which will represent 38 percent of its total energy, notes Rich.
Another project captures flaring methane gas from the La Crosse City
Brewery to convert the beer maker's wasted biogas discharge into some
2 million kilowatt hours per year of electricity—about 2 percent of the

system's energy goal. Similarly, on its campus in Onalaska, yet another program captures methane from a nearby La Crosse County landfill and pipes it under a highway to generators on the hospital grounds, transforming it into electricity, some of which is sold back to the county. That project enabled facility managers at the Onalaska campus to shut down boilers for two large buildings totaling 340,000 square feet and draw all energy for heat and hot water from the new project. Excess power is being pushed onto the power grid.

Then there's the poop-power project. Gunderson is teaming up with three farm families and Dane County to build the county's second manure digester, which will convert cow manure to renewable gas energy. A local utility will purchase the 11,000 kilowatt hours of electricity generated by the project, enough to power about 1,600 homes. As a co-benefit, the project will further the county's efforts to reduce phosphorus runoff into its waterways. And, says Rich, the byproduct from the digesters can be turned into composted soil amendment or potting soil, which can be sold. He says the project will account for 9 percent of Gunderson's energy goal.

Finally, Gunderson is in the early stages of building a new 400,000-square foot hospital and retrofitting existing facilities. All new construction is being designed to achieve LEED certification, incorporating design features to keep future energy needs at a minimum. For example, close attention was paid to where windows face to maximize exposure to heat from the sun. And a geothermal system was installed for non–fossil fuel heating and cooling.

Rich estimates that Gundersen's entire energy program will have an estimated 7-year rate of return on investment. They are optimistic they will achieve their goal of independence from fossil fuels by the 2014 target date. The program has been so successful and garnered so much interest from other hospitals that Envision is creating a separate consultancy division to help others with energy audits and offer advice on setting goals for energy independence.

Rich attributes Gundersen's remarkable achievements and its culture of sustainability to two factors: intense focus and leadership. "We gave ourselves a fairly short timeline to accomplish this goal. If you give yourself a goal, it shouldn't take twenty years because then there's no urgency. You lose constancy of purpose if it takes too long. Also, our CEO is the number one champion behind sustainability. He encourages us to take risks and challenge ourselves beyond what's normally expected. He tells us to have courage and then make reasonable decisions and do the right thing from a stewardship perspective.[36]

According to CEO Dr. Thompson, "We can improve the health of the communities we serve and reduce the cost of care with savings generated from our sustainability program. For us, it was never a question of why would we develop a program like this. It's a question of: why wouldn't we?"[37]

Case Studies: More Low-Cost, High-Impact Approaches to Energy Freedom

Gundersen Lutheran's story has certainly raised the bar for all health systems working to reduce their contributions to climate change and its health impacts. There have been scores of innovative and inspiring, if less noticed, climate-related initiatives at large and small health systems across the nation in recent years. Few examples are as all-encompassing as Gundersen, but several have achieved remarkable gains against greenhouse gas emissions while improving health care. And many of these programs do not require costly installation of solar panels, wind turbines, cogeneration equipment, fuel cells, biomass boilers, or manure digesters.

Patient-Centered Lighting at Cleveland Clinic
As noted previously, something as relatively simple as substituting compact fluorescent and light-emitting diodes (LEDs) for incandescent light bulbs can result in huge energy savings and reductions in heat. Improved management of campus-wide lighting was one of the important ways that the Cleveland Clinic achieved the US EPA's coveted Energy Star Partner of the Year award 2 years in a row. John L. D'Angelo, the former senior

director for facilities at Cleveland Clinic, attributes their impressive energy efficiency accomplishments to the fact that they do not even refer to their approach as an energy efficiency program.[38]

"We don't have an energy program and never will," asserts D'Angelo. "It's a patient-centered program. My job is 100 percent focused on patient outcomes, safety and experience. We tied all of our support functions to those three critical missions, including how we use our energy. By intelligently using our energy, we can positively affect patient outcomes. By having better maintenance of our HVAC, we are reducing hospital acquired infections. More efficient equipment has created a significant amount of energy savings, but that wasn't the reason we did it."

The clinic's substitution of more than 60,000 LED bulbs for nearly all the incandescent lights is a case in point. "LED lighting reduces the load on the wiring, which reduces the chance of fire," says D'Angelo. And since LEDs emit less energy than incandescents, "it also reduces the load on the building transformers, which reduces chances for an outage that could affect patient care. They also free up more space on the emergency generators so if there is an outage, more things can get powered for us to keep operating."

Dimmed nighttime lighting, he says, addresses a perennial problem that patients often complain about: the difficulty of getting a good night's sleep in a hospital due to noisy staff during shift changes. By dimming corridor lights at night to the egress minimums, they created a hushed atmosphere that encouraged staff to talk more quietly.

"Our patient satisfaction numbers have gone up since then, and the side benefit is we're using less energy for lighting." What's more, the lighting changes resulted in the Cleveland Clinic saving about $4 million in energy costs per year, for a total of almost $20 million in a 4-year period, says D'Angelo.

Tapping Landfill Gas for Energy at Dignity Health's Marian Medical Center

Dignity Health created a notable program focused on using renewable energy and reducing GHGs at its Marian Medical Center in Santa Maria, California. Through the partnership with a local landfill, the medical center was able to use landfill gas as a fuel source for energy. Two miles of pipes were laid to pump the landfill gas onsite and feed a 1-megawatt generator, fulfilling close to 95 percent of the medical center's energy needs.

Through the use of this sustainable long-term renewable energy source, the hospital has been able to save $300,000 per year and avoid the equivalent of more than 42,000 tons of carbon dioxide per year. Future plans include a 1.4-megawatt expansion, which will use waste heat from the engine generators to supply steam and hot water to the hospital to curtail additional energy use requirements.[39]

COMPUTER PURCHASING AND DATA CENTER EFFICIENCY AT KAISER PERMANENTE

Other low-cost, high-impact strategies involve purchasing decisions, especially around energy-intense products like computers and printers. Kaiser Permanente changed 98 percent of our printer equipment to Energy Star products and set the default to double-sided printing. That reduced energy demand by 3,600-kilowatt hours and saved 240 million sheets of paper for a total dollar savings of $7 million annually.[40]

In 2006, we began a transition to computers that adhere to the Electronic Product Environmental Assessment Tool (EPEAT) certification tool. This fulfilled most of the criteria we wanted whenever we purchased new equipment: the least possible toxic materials (such as cadmium and mercury), designed for easy recycling, minimal energy demand, and minimal packaging materials. Between 2006 and 2011, we purchased more than 60,000 computers, 66,000 monitors, and nearly 9,000 notebook computers. Our purchasing of EPEAT-registered computers has risen from around 45 percent to 99.5 percent of all EPEAT-eligible laptops, desktops, and monitors, with 78 percent meeting the top-level EPEAT-Gold certification. The result has been vast reductions in toxic materials, a decrease in energy use, and energy savings of $4 million to $5 million annually, all at no additional purchasing cost.[41]

Even greater energy reductions have come from innovative energy-saving strategies at our five national data centers, which have been experiencing a doubling every year in data storage requirements. Steven Press, executive director of Data Center Facilities Services at Kaiser Permanente, created "Keep IT Green" teams at the centers to develop ideas about energy savings and share ideas with the data center industry.

Measuring energy use in the data centers has proven essential, says Press. His teams developed a method capturing all energy use information and fine-tuning the computer rooms at a highly granular level. That effort resulted in avoidance of 450 million kilowatts of electricity required annually at one data center. Along with other initiatives in that state-of-the-art center, they avoided $700,000 of annual operating costs in 2011 and expect to continue reaping those savings going forward. As an added bonus, the data center received a US EPA Energy Star award and became the first data center to be awarded LEED Platinum certification for operations and maintenance in an existing building.

"We continue to take these learnings and use them across our entire portfolio and in new designs," says Press. "In data centers we have to continue to update the mechanical and electrical systems. Every time we do that we bring in the most efficient system available."[42] Over the most recent years, the focus on energy efficiency, he adds, has avoided 2 megawatts of energy demand and eliminated the need to build two more data centers.

TRANSPORTATION AT SEATTLE CHILDREN'S HOSPITAL

Another major source for reduction of GHG emissions is transportation. According to the US EPA, 27 percent of GHG emissions in the United States came from transportation sources in 2008, thus not only contributing to climate change but also—owing to the harmful co-pollutants that result from combusting fossil fuels—reducing local air quality, which directly impacts people with heart or respiratory disease. The Seattle Children's Hospital recently decided to target employee and visitor use of single-occupancy vehicles as part of a comprehensive, $4 million transportation management plan that focuses on the health and environmental benefits of cycling, walking, using public transit, and even intelligent transportation system software that reduces vehicle delays and travel time at key local intersections. The plan includes shuttle-to-transit systems linking the hospital to regional transit hubs and financial incentives for employees who commute without driving alone. They are even offering, among numerous other features, a shared bike program and free bicycles to employees committed to cycling at least 2 days per week. Since its inception, the hospital's alternative commuting efforts have taken 630,000 car trips off the roads and freeways, reduced vehicle miles traveled by 6.5 million miles, and saved 235,000 gallons of gasoline.[43]

Virtual Office Visits at Kaiser Permanente

Kaiser Permanente has promoted a number of transportation-related efficiencies over the years, but one of the more surprising results came from a technology that at first glance seems totally unconnected with transportation. It is the system's state-of-the-art electronic medical record system, known as KP Health Connect and its associated Web-based member interface known as My Health Manager. By using My Health Manager, health plan members can order prescriptions, make appointments, and even ask questions of their doctors and get prompt replies. While the technology was implemented primarily to improve patient care and service, it has produced a number of co-benefits for our sustainability efforts, including avoidance of auto emissions. A published analysis by Kaiser Permanente researchers shows that the use of the technology accomplished the following climate benefits in a single year:

- Eliminated up to 92,000 tons of carbon dioxide emissions associated with transportation by replacing face-to-face doctor–patient visits with virtual online visits.
- Avoided 7,000 tons of carbon dioxide emissions by enabling members to fill their prescription medications online and by mail delivery.
- Resulted in a positive net effect on the environment despite increased energy use and additional waste from the greater use of personal computers.[44]

The aforementioned examples only begin to suggest the number of innovative and effective, and often surprising, ways that health care systems are dealing with the health challenges of climate change. These and other organizations are devising, implementing, and sharing a host of additional strategies to reduce greenhouse emissions through both radical and incremental changes. Incorporating evidence-based, green design principles and carbon-absorbing landscaping into tomorrow's hospital campuses can, if practiced widely, bring American health care ever closer to a zero-carbon footprint. The growing number of health systems signing on to Health Care Without Harm's Healthy Food Pledge and setting targets for local and sustainable food purchasing is avoiding the use of pesticides and fertilizers that are typically made from fossil fuels. Even efforts to reduce or eliminate the use of single-use bottled water in favor of filtered tap water in hospitals can have a surprisingly large impact on GHG emissions, as do the growing number of effective solid waste management options that health systems have developed.

In the following chapters, I will explore how changes in all of these domains—food services, waste management, management of harmful chemicals and toxins, and green hospital design—can not only mitigate many of the threatened health impacts of a warming world and a changing climate but can also serve the broader goals of environmental and health care sustainability.

NOTES

1. Intergovernmental Panel on Climate Change, "Climate Change 2007: Synthesis Report," http://www.ipcc.ch/publications_and_data/ar4/syr/en/mains6-1.html.
2. IPCC Working Group, "Climate Change 2013: The Physical Science Basis, Summary for Policymakers," November 2013, http://www.climate2013.org/spm.
3. Ibid.
4. A. Costello, M. Abbas, A. Allen, et al., "Managing the Health Effects of Climate Change." *Lancet* 373, no. 9676 (2009): 1693–1733.
5. National Research Council, *Advancing the Science of Climate Change* (Washington, DC: National Academies Press, 2010).
6. "Climate Change: The Biggest Global-Health Threat of the 21st Century," *University College London News*, May 14, 2009, http://www.ucl.ac.uk/news/news-articles/0905/09051501.

7. World Medical Association, "Doctors' Leader Criticises Governments for Paying Poor Attention to Heath in Climate Change Debate," October 16, 2009, http://www.wma.net/en/40news/20archives/2009/2009_11/.

8. Perry E. Sheffield and Philip J. Landrigan, "Global Climate Change and Children's Health: Threats and Strategies for Prevention," *Environmental Health Perspectives* 119, no. 3 (March 2011): 291–298.

9. US EPA, "Climate Impacts on Human Health," http://www.epa.gov/climatechange/impacts-adaptation/health.html.

10. US Global Change Research Program, "Global Climate Change Impacts in the US: Executive Summary," http://downloads.globalchange.gov/usimpacts/pdfs/executive-summary.pdf.

11. US EPA, "Climate Change Indicators in the United States," http://www.epa.gov/climatechange/science/indicators/weather-climate/precipitation.html.

12. Ibid.

13. US EPA, "Combined Sewer Overflows Demographics," http://cfpub.epa.gov/npdes/cso/demo.cfm.

14. A. Nagourney, I. Lovett, "Severe Drought Has U.S. West Fearing Worst," *New York Times*, February 1, 2014.

15. Bradford H. Gray and Kathy Hebert, "After Katrina" (Urban Institute, July 2006).

16. J. David Goodman and Colin Moynihan, "Patients Evacuated from City Medical Center after Power Failure," *New York Times*, October 30, 2012.

17. Spivey Lipsey, interviewed by Judith Nemes, 2011.

18. John Messervy, interviewed by Judith Nemes, 2011–2012.

19. American Lung Association, Key Findings for 2009–2011, http://www.stateoftheair.org/2013/key-findings/.

20. California Air Resources Board, *Recent Research Findings: Health Effects of Particulate Matter and Ozone Air Pollution*, online face sheet, 2007, http://www.arb.ca.gov/research/health/healthres.htm#6pm.

21. "Global Climate Change Impacts in the US."

22. US CDC, "West Nile Virus," http://www.cdc.gov/ncidod/dvbid/westnile/index.htm.

23. Diarmid Campbell-Lendrum, Carlos Corvalán, and Maria Neira, "Global Climate Change: Implications for International Public Health Policy," *Bulletin of the World Health Organization* 85, no. 3 (March 2007): 161–244.

24. Ibid.

25. Dylan Walsh, "The Baffling Nexus of Climate Change and Health," *New York Times*, September 6, 2012.

26. Trust for America's Health and the Robert Woods Johnson Foundation, "Outbreaks: Protection Americans from Disease," http://www.healthyamericans.org/assets/files/TFAH2013OutbreaksRpt07.pdf

27. Ceres, "Insurer Climate Risk Disclosure Survey 2012," March 7, 2013, http://www.ceres.org/resources/reports/naic-report/view.

28. US Energy Information Agency, "Commercial Buildings Energy Consumption Survey, Energy Characteristics and Energy Consumed in Large Hospital Buildings in 2007," August 17, 2012, http://www.eia.gov/consumption/commercial/reports/2007/large-hospital.cfm.

29. Jeanette Chung, "Estimate of the Carbon Footprint of the US Health Care Sector," *JAMA* 302, no. 18 (November 11, 2009): 1970–1972.

30. Environment Science Center, "Greener Hospitals: Improving Environmental Performance," 11, http://www.bms.com/Documents/sustainability/downloads/greenh.pdf.

31. Hina Gadani and Arun Vyas, "Anesthetic Gases and Global Warming: Potentials, Prevention, and Future of Anesthesia," *Anesthesia Essays and Researches* 5, no. 1 (2011): 5–10.

32. The Lund Report, "Kaiser Permanente Pledges Major Reduction in Greenhouse Gases," February 29, 2012, http://www.thelundreport.org/resource/kaiser_permanente_pledges_major_reduction_in_greenhouse_gases?page=3.

33. Kaiser Permanente, "Kaiser Permanente Cuts Electricity Use in Parking Garage at New Westside Medical Center," press release, September 11, 2012, http://share.kaiserpermanente.org/article/kaiser-permanente-cuts-electricity-use-in-parking-garage-at-new-westside-medical-center.

34. Jeff Rich, interviewed by Judith Nemes, 2011.

35. Jessica Larsen, "Wisconsin's First Community Wind Farm Up and Running in Cashton," *LaCrosse Tribune*, July 18, 2012.

36. Rich interviewed by Nemes.

37. Bob Herman, "How Gundersen Lutheran Health System Will Be Energy Independent by 2014," *Beckers's Hospital Review*, June 11, 2012.

38. John L. D'Angelo, interviewed by Judith Nemes.

39. Healthier Hospitals, "Case Study: Dignity Health—Renewable Energy at Marin Medical Center," http://healthierhospitals.org/sites/default/files/IMCE/public_files/Case_Study_Images/Marin%20Medical.pdf.

40. John Ebers, presentation at the ACCO Healthy Hospitals Workshop, Chicago, June 13, 2011.

41. Healthier Hospitals Initiative "Case Study Kaiser Permanente: Electronic Products Environmental Assessment Tool (EPEAT)—Purchasing Environmentally Responsible Computers, April 2, 2012.

42. Steve Press, interviewed by Judith Nemes.

43. Janet Brown, "Conscious Commuting: A Look into the Comprehensive Transportation Plan Developed at Seattle Children's Hospital," *Healthcare Design*, March 1, 2011, http://www.healthcaredesignmagazine.com/article/conscious-commuting-look-comprehensive-transportation-plan-developed-seattle-childrens-hospi.

44. Marianne Turley et al., "Use of Electronic Health Records Can Improve the Health Care Industry's Environmental Footprint," *Health Affairs* 30, no. 5 (May 2011): 938–946.

3

The Business Case for Total Health

Can environmental sustainability strategies in health care coexist with today's constant pressures on cost structures? For many health care organizations, that question lies at the heart of the viability of the greening of health care movement. Is it affordable? How do we tally the costs and benefits?

Fortunately, there is a preponderance of evidence that a greener health care enterprise is not only affordable but that in most cases it results in an improved cost structure. The latest comprehensive examination of the question estimates that if the health care industry conserved energy, reduced waste, and more efficiently purchased operating supplies, it could save more than $15 billion over 10 years.[1]

Efforts by hospitals to develop greener, more environmentally sustainable operations result in significant savings rather than incur additional costs, according to the study of nine hospitals/health systems that undertook a range of initiatives, including improvements in waste management, energy reduction, and operating room supply procurement, over a 5-year period. The study's authors concluded that if similar changes were adopted throughout the US health care sector, the total savings could exceed $5.4 billion over 5 years, and $15 billion over 10 years.

"This study turns on its head the belief that introducing environmental sustainability measures increases operating costs," said Blair L. Sadler, JD, senior fellow at the Institute for Healthcare Improvement, one of the study authors, and former CEO of Rady Children's Hospital, San Diego, California. "In fact, it is just the opposite," he says. "With little or no capital investments, significant operating savings can be realized. It is good for patients and staff, and is a better strategy than having to lay off valuable personnel or closing effective programs that lose money."[2]

From 2009 to 2012, Kaiser Permanente pursued environmentally preferable product and service contracts have yielded savings of $63 million. Our contract savings often result from standardization and efficiencies by our expert procurement team, and they do not always reflect a less expensive product.

In the beginning of Kaiser Permanente's environmental stewardship efforts, our cost structure was less of a driver than our health care mission, so long as our program was cost neutral in the long run. Actually, what we had in the early days was not so much a stewardship "program" as a shared understanding about the link between environmental health and human health and a belief that, as a major health care provider, we had a great opportunity, and a responsibility, to act on that link. We understood that the health and sustainability of the environment—the natural environment, the built environment, and even the social environment—is a necessary condition for human health and well-being. We think of our mission in terms of what we call "total health," which has multiple, interrelated dimensions. It includes the physical, emotional, and spiritual health of every individual, supported and sustained by the health of our total environment—our families, neighborhoods, workplaces, cities, the air we breathe, the food and water we consume, and all the delicate ecological balances that sustain life on this planet. While medical care is typically focused on the physical health of patients and members, our approach to health and wellness must support this larger reality.

Besides this shared ethos, we also had organizational leadership that was deeply committed to the total health vision and designated a single point person (which turned out to be me) to identify and coordinate the various green projects that were sprouting throughout the organization into a more focused and strategic effort. From the beginning, we took a "distributed accountability" approach to the work. We embedded environmental stewardship into the operations of the organization and created an Environmental Stewardship Council. We had three priority areas: sustainable purchasing, sustainable operations, and sustainable buildings. The operations team agreed on a plan to prioritize waste reduction—one of the lowest hanging fruits in health care—as our first major project. We formed the Waste Minimization Team, and we developed a toolkit that our hospital managers could use to conduct waste assessments. It demonstrated the potential savings and environmental benefits that could result from something as simple as segregating regular trash, which costs about 3 to 8 cents a pound to process, from biohazardous and regulated medical waste, which costs up to $2 per pound to process. At the same time, we also acted on the emerging evidence about the hazardous nature of polyvinyl chlorides (PVCs) by working to remove PVC-containing materials from the waste stream.

From there, we moved quickly to the elimination of mercury, a powerful neurotoxin. While hospitals were not the main source of mercury pollution, the incineration of medical wastes nonetheless contributed nearly 16 tons of the toxin into the atmosphere every year, about 10 percent of all the nation's mercury air emissions.[3] In the atmosphere, it could travel anywhere from a few hundred feet to thousands of miles away from its original source, making it possible for an incinerator in Nebraska to contaminate cod in the Atlantic.

Eliminating mercury taught us the value of evaluating products on the basis of "total cost of ownership." A unit-by-unit cost comparison showed that most alternatives to mercury-containing devices, such as electronic, battery-operated thermometers, were more expensive than the mercury-containing devices that our hospitals already owned. In the end, we were able to show that the combined cost of spill kits and the expense of closing down an exam room after a mercury spill—an infrequent but not a rare event—was in fact much higher than switching to mercury-free devices. We documented that when hazardous waste disposal, staff training, and the like are taken into account, the total cost of ownership per unit of a mercury-free blood pressure device is about one third that of a mercury-containing device.

Within a few years, digital thermometers were the norm throughout our hospitals and clinics, and all purchases of new blood pressure cuffs were required to be mercury-free. We also implemented recycling of all the mercury in fluorescent bulbs and required our vendors to itemize any mercury in their products and to provide nontoxic alternatives. By 2008, Kaiser Permanente was virtually mercury-free, along with a growing number of other health systems that had signed on to Health Care Without Harm's Mercury-Free Pledge. In 2007, the estimated cost savings to our organization in avoiding mercury safety equipment, which included mercury cleanup kits and special vacuums, was $500,000. Other cost savings included reduced hazardous spill cleanup costs (at least $2,500 each) and uncalculated costs of clinic closure due to a spill.

The success of those first two projects, waste minimization and eliminating mercury-containing devices, clearly demonstrated that we could achieve significant environmental benefits while also making our facilities safer for our patients and our employees. And we could save money—or at least not create new costs—in the bargain. In fact, those three objectives—patient and staff health and safety, responsible environmental stewardship, and cost savings—became the principal criteria by which we evaluated all future ideas. Any proposal that met all three criteria shot to the top of our project list. Even if some projects, such as switching to safer cleaning products, involved short-term excess costs, those would make the agenda, as well, so long as they delivered significant health and environmental benefits that in the long run would make them cost-effective.

The Triple Bottom Line

Our three requirements for taking on a green project turned out to be closely in tune with thinking that was emerging among environmental activists, economists, biologists, and future-oriented entrepreneurs about the sustainability of living systems and the laws that govern commercial economic activity. Over the next decade, these ideas would have a major impact on attitudes about how businesses of all kinds define successful performance, as well as the responsibilities that organizations bear toward their shareholders and stakeholders.

The concepts developed and popularized have come to constitute a persuasive and widely embraced rationale, or business case, for the greening of business operations, in investor-owned and nonprofit entities, and for the broader movement of environmental sustainability that links humanity's social and economic well-being to the long-term resilience of life on earth. The arguments provided are worth examining, at least briefly, for they answer the question of why a growing vanguard of large and small businesses, nonprofits, and even governments have embraced values, beliefs, and codes of conduct that would have been almost unthinkable in most executive suites less than two decades ago.

Our business case for greening projects—the health of our patients, staff, and communities; the health of the environment, locally and globally; and our financial health—was not fundamentally different from an emerging theory known as the "triple bottom line." This is a concept first articulated in 1994 by John Elkington, the founder of a British consulting firm called Sustain Ability, who expanded on the theory in his book *Cannibals with Forks: The Triple Bottom Line of 21st Century Business.*[4] Elkington proposed that in an era of increasingly constrained natural resources and growing environmental degradation, a new framework was needed to measure the performance of a business or an entire economy that could look beyond the traditional bottom line of profitability and return on investment to include environmental and social costs and benefits. Only by measuring and accounting for the total sum of the interrelated investments and outcomes along the dimensions of people, profit, and planet—the 3Ps—could an enterprise evaluate its true-cost performance and sustainability. The triple bottom line concept, says business writer Andrew Savitz, "captures the essence of sustainability by measuring the impact of an organization's activities on the world...including both its profitability and shareholder values and its social, human, and environmental capital."[5]

The addition of social and environmental capital to the financial balance sheet was an important acknowledgment that, just as all types of businesses depends on financial capital in the form of investments and equipment, they also depend on the capital, or services, provided by a healthy society and a healthy environment. Social capital comes in the form of loyal, skilled employees; supportive communities; loyal customers; suppliers; investors; and the legal and governmental institutions of civil society. The environment contributes sources of energy, forests for wood products, arable land for agriculture, clean air and plentiful clean water, minerals, chemicals, plants and animals, and the like. Basically, healthy societies and environments provide the raw materials for virtually all the services and goods of the consumer society, in addition to protection from the sun's radiation, medicines, recycling of wastes, erosion control, and a host of other natural services that sustain life on earth and enable economic growth.

To ignore the value of this social and environmental capital in the overall performance of a business, a government, or a nonprofit organization is to court bankruptcy, because what we do not assign a true value to we are prone to take for granted and waste. In the case of critical natural resources, we have been spending down vast sums of nonrenewable capital for generations. The US Environmental Protection Agency (EPA) reports that humans have consumed more natural resources in the last 50 years than in all previous history. A century ago, 41 percent of the raw materials used in the United States were renewable (agriculture, fisheries, and forest products). By the end of the twentieth century, only 6 percent of the materials we consumed were renewable; the rest consisted of finite resources, such as minerals, metals, and products derived from fossil fuels.[6]

As the environmental writer and business entrepreneur Paul Hawken put it in an influential article, "Commercial institutions do not see that healthy living systems—clean air and water, healthy soil, stable climates— are integral to a functioning economy. As our living systems deteriorate, traditional forecasting and business economics become the equivalent of house rules on a sinking ship."[7]

Over the past 15 years, the triple bottom line framework and its implications have served as powerful drivers behind a major shift in the strategic outlook of a growing number of commercial enterprises, including nonprofits for which bottom line profitability, or return on investment (ROI), was never the sole arbiter of success. The embrace of sustainability as a business model has been such that an entire industry has grown up around the ranking of the "sustainability performance" of companies, led by the Dow Jones Sustainability Index, launched in 1999. It evaluates the largest 2,500 companies listed on the Dow Jones for specific measures of their financial, social, and environmental operations. Its annual rankings have become the key reference point for another industry, that of sustainability or corporate responsibility investing, in which investors seek out companies with high scores in assessments of economic, social, and environmental asset management as the best candidates for long-term profitability and sustainability.

As John Prestbo, the president of Dow Jones Indexes, says, "Sustainability has become a proxy for enlightened and disciplined management, which just happens to be the most important factor that investors do and should consider in deciding where to buy a stock."[8]

IT'S ALL ABOUT HEALTH

But what about health care, an industry that many would argue is fundamentally different from either the normal Main Street or Wall Street models of capitalist enterprise? Can the same sort of accounting standards apply?

Roughly 60 percent of all hospitals in the United States today, and 86 percent of all "hospital assets," are nonprofit—a share that has been declining for several decades.[9] But this does not mean that the health care sector does not need to focus on the bottom line, which nonprofits define as "margin" rather than profit. Nonprofit health care executives often quote the phrase "no margin, no mission" to emphasize the fact that if costs exceed revenues, the organization's social mission is likely to suffer. Most nonprofit health care organizations have a mission statement that commits them to providing high-quality care to their community of

patients at affordable costs. Every year nonprofit health care organizations are required to provide extensive evidence to the Internal Revenue
Service that they are fulfilling that mission. If they fail the test, they can,
and do, lose their nonprofit status.

Kaiser Permanente's mission is to "provide high-quality, affordable
health care services and to improve the health of our members and the
communities we serve"—a statement that many of the organization's physicians and employees know by heart and that truly drives the culture of
the organization. But we also understand that over time we need to generate more revenue than we incur in costs—a margin—if we are to fulfill
our responsibilities to our "shareholders," which in our case includes our
9.1 million dues-paying members *and* the far-larger populations of the
communities in which we operate.

We care about margin because it goes directly to fulfilling our mission, the
health of our members and our communities. As former Kaiser Permanente
Chairman and CEO David Lawrence told one of the earliest conferences on
green health care back in 2000, "We all know the old saw 'no margin, no
mission.' But…without the mission, I don't want to get up in the morning.
Competing effectively is a need that we all have, but it isn't what health care
is about. It's about improving the health of the communities we serve."[10]

Thus, while the triple bottom line is clearly relevant to health care, in
our formulation it describes a business case with a difference. Instead of
the equally weighted 3Ps of people, profit, and planet, we aim to achieve
a primary bottom line of what we call "total health." By that we mean the
integrated health of people's bodies, minds, and spirits, achieved through
activities and services that contribute to healthy populations and healthy
communities, all of which ultimately depend on healthy environments—
and, yes, healthy margins to sustain and improve the services. As Ray
Baxter, PhD, senior vice president of Community Benefit, Research, and
Health Policy at Kaiser Permanente, often reminds us, the agendas for our
environmental stewardship program and our related community benefit
activities—programs in which we have invested close to $2 billion annu-
ally in recent years—are not primarily about saving the planet, achieving
social equity, or saving money. "We need to be clear that everything we do

is anchored to health, because that's where our credibility is, and that's what our mission is."[11] The point is that all of our efforts in environmental stewardship are ultimately about improving the health of our communities.

Or, as Loel Solomon, vice president for community health at Kaiser Permanente, puts it, "We come at our environmental work from a health perspective, not because it's the green thing to do. The same strategies that reduce toxicity in our environment and carbon dioxide emissions and conserve energy are the same strategies that reduce illness in our society and reduce society's health care costs."[12]

This broad definition of health, directly linking the total health of the individual to social and environmental health, has had the advantage of forcing us to connect the dots of what used to be relatively siloed streams of work throughout the organization—medical care in our hospitals and clinics, one-off environmental projects both inside and outside the hospitals' walls, and community benefit work in schools, workplaces, safety net clinics, and elsewhere (see Fig. 3.1). The result is a more focused, integrated vision and strategy in which every area of work benefits from its relationship to the rest. Our environmental stewardship agenda is therefore prioritized and shaped by how it can leverage other work streams to have the greatest impact on the health of our members and our communities.

Robert Pearl, MD, who heads The Permanente Medical Group—the large physician group that provides all the care for Kaiser Permanente's 3.4 million members in Northern California—argues that having such

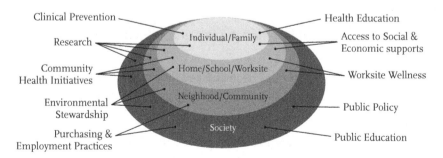

Figure 3.1
Total Health at Kaiser Permanente. Promoting clinical, educational, environmental, and social actions to improve health.

a big-picture strategy allows leaders to focus on "how the pieces come together, not just whether solar panels are too expensive to buy today, or whether or not to get rid of all mercury." Pearl, who also teaches a course on strategy at the Stanford Graduate School of Business, adds, "The business case for environmental stewardship is massive, but you have to stop asking 'Does this piece, alone, make sense? Because, in the end, all the pieces have to work together. Having a comprehensive strategy allows us to make difficult decisions in ambiguous circumstances. It allows us to make the choice that is environmentally sustainable because it aligns to our values and our mission."[13]

A health-centered approach to environmental activities has spread far and wide in the health care sector. At one of the early major medical profession workshops on the greening of health care, sponsored by the Institute of Medicine, Howard Frumkin, MD, then director of the National Center for Environmental Health at the US Centers for Disease Control and Prevention (CDC), summed up the key motives that drive health systems and health professionals to embrace environmental stewardship: It appeals, he said, to physicians' traditional ethics relating to beneficence, non-maleficence, and justice; it contributes to increased market share; it promotes the well-being of communities and allows health care institutions to demonstrate community leadership; it saves money; and so on. But for the health professionals attending the conference, he said, the most compelling case for green health care was simply "its potential to protect and promote health."[14]

Environmental Stewardship and the Prevention Paradigm

While the health mission has been the key driver in the rapid growth of green health care from the fringes of the industry to the mainstream, that mission can never be separated from the social and economic missions. The three bottom lines are inextricably linked. As noted in the first two chapters, a large and growing body of scientific evidence over the last two decades has linked environmental factors to rapidly rising rates of costly and debilitating chronic diseases. An equally impressive body of evidence links many of these same chronic conditions to socioeconomic factors, including education, income, neighborhood characteristics, and ethnic and racial background. Until these "upstream" determinants of health are fully recognized and addressed throughout the health care sector, the escalating incidence and cost of these diseases will remain a direct threat not only to the nation's health but to its wealth as well.

Fortunately, a consensus already exists among health professionals that the focus of health care delivery needs to shift from the traditional and prevailing model of treating acute conditions—those that most often land people in emergency rooms and hospital beds, such as heart attacks and strokes—to one focused more broadly on preventive care and the upstream social, behavioral, genetic, and environmental causes of disease, including the contributors to obesity, respiratory illness, and developmental disorders. Medical care alone is now understood to be a relatively less significant factor among the total determinants of health than these upstream contributors, as shown in Figure 3.2.

Even today, powerful economic incentives created as part of the 2010 federal health reform law, the Affordable Care Act, along with the

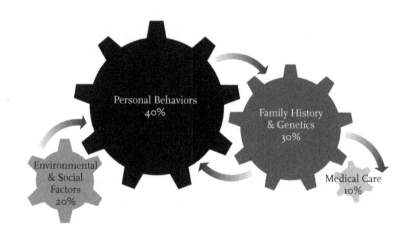

Figure 3.2
Drivers of health.
(source: The Case for More Active Policy Attention to Health Promotion, J. Michael McGinnis, Pamela Williams-Russo, and James R. Knickman, *Health Affairs* 27 no. 2 (March 2002): 78–93.)

examples provided by some of the nation's top-quality health care providers, have been leading the health care mainstream in this new direction. The prevention model focuses on better early diagnosis and management of chronic, long-term health conditions like diabetes and asthma and a strategy that seeks to reduce the incidence of chronic conditions (along with the acute health problems that result from them) through individual and social behavioral changes and changes in those environmental factors known to be linked to human health.

A recent study by scientists at the CDC quantified the health and cost benefits of this prevention/environmental health approach.[15] Using a simulation model of the entire US health care system, scientists compared three health care strategies for reducing total US mortality and improving costs. One strategy was to extend health care coverage to all Americans through a universal care program similar to the 2010 Affordable Care Act, which aims to reduce costly health care utilization by providing near-universal access to primary and secondary care and preventive services—basically, provide effective and timely care more broadly to reduce the costs of neglected care. The second strategy, improved care, focused on delivering better, more consistent disease screening and chronic care management, including more consistent patient and physician adherence to evidence-based care guidelines. The final strategy emphasized interventions that promote healthier personal and social behaviors, such as smoking cessation, healthy eating, and greater physical activity, along with activities to promote safer, healthier environments that reduce the prevalence of avoidable, environmentally linked diseases.

The CDC analysts concluded that each of the three strategies could cost-effectively save tens of thousands of lives annually, though they would be far more effective if implemented in combination. While the first two strategies, universal coverage and improved screening and chronic care management, initially would be more effective at saving lives, they also would tend to increase costs the most because they would increase the use of constrained health resources, such as primary care providers. Only the behavioral and environmental protection strategy, they concluded, would, over a 10- to 25-year period, save more lives at lower costs due to its ability to slow the prevalence of diseases without creating new demands on primary care capacity. When added to the first two strategies, the prevention/environmental approach "could save 90 percent more lives and reduce costs by 30 percent" within 10 years.

For hospital systems that struggle to maintain margins of just 2 to 4 percent, the combination of lives saved and costs avoided constitutes a compelling business case for an aggressive, prevention-oriented environmental stewardship strategy.

CHALLENGING THE COST MYTH

Environmental interventions that both promote better health and have a positive or neutral impact on hospital budgets are a double winner: They save lives and make health care more affordable for everyone. Much of the conventional wisdom about the increased cost of environmental safeguards, green-designed hospitals, substitution of toxic products and chemicals, and alternative, more efficient energy systems has been proven wrong.

Although green alternatives to standard products sometimes have higher initial costs, a different picture emerges when one looks at the total, lifetime cost of ownership of a hospital, a product, or a technology. Like the elimination of mercury, the initial cost of alternative devices was somewhat greater, but the lifetime cost, including the avoided cost of staff training and special spill cleanup supplies, made the alternatives not only safer but less expensive. Had that not been the case, mercury thermometers might well still be ubiquitous in hospitals today instead of having virtually disappeared.

The same calculus applies across a broad range of environmental mitigation strategies, from simple waste recycling to the design and construction of sustainable facilities. In fact, our efforts to identify and purchase environmentally safer, nontoxic products and services from 2009 through 2012 resulted in $63 million in savings for Kaiser Permanente. We did not purchase those products to save that money; we did it to provide safer, more effective health care. But we applied sound procurement efficiencies, standardized product lines, and calculated the total cost of ownership in order to achieve cost savings.

The cost effectiveness of environmental stewardship in health care is particularly strong for new facilities, especially when energy conservation and toxic-free materials are built into the design. Architect John Kouletsis, Kaiser Permanente's VP of facilities planning, says that "we find that if we approach hospital design from an environmental and patient safety perspective, we don't really increase our capital cost structure. We make sure that any addition from a sustainability standpoint has to have a return on investment in 3–4 years. What we discovered is that those investments are either neutral or cheaper over the life of the asset compared to other things we might have done."[16]

A True Fable of Green Hospitals

The business case for green health care has rarely been more persuasively demonstrated than in the case of the Fable Hospital, a brand new 300-bed, 600,000-square foot regional medical center built at a cost of $350 million in 2011. Fable was designed and constructed to meet the US Green Building Council's Leadership in Energy and Environmental Design (LEED) gold-certification level for green building design, construction, operations, and maintenance. To do so, it included the best innovations for which there was strong evidence in the scientific literature that they would improve patient and employee safety and health care quality while also reducing operating (but not initial construction) costs. Every single attribute of the design had been thoroughly evaluated in other new or remodeled hospitals for its impact on the health of patients, families, staff, and, where applicable, the environment. These included such features as larger single-patient, acuity-adaptable rooms to reduce incidents of health care–associated infections and patient transfers; use of nontoxic building materials to reduce the effects of indoor air pollution; high-efficiency particulate air (HEPA) filtration systems that remove 99.97 percent of all particles greater than 0.3 micrometers from the air; larger windows to increase the beneficial effects of natural light and nature views; single-use air circulation systems to minimize the spread of infections; heat recovery systems, high-efficiency mechanical equipment, and external building glazing to reduce fossil fuel consumption; healing gardens accessible by patients and staff; low-flow water fixtures and rainwater recapture systems to reduce water consumption; and dozens of other features.

The Fable Hospital, as you might guess, is a fable, constructed in an essay by health care quality experts from the US CDC and assisted by the staff at the Center for Health Design.[17] But the imaginary hospital they conceived represented an amalgamation of innovative quality and environmental features that had been implemented and evaluated in real hospitals with the help of the Center for Health Design's Pebble Project. That project is a research initiative dedicated to designing, measuring, and documenting the outcomes of innovations in hospital safety, clinical quality, environmental performance, and operating efficiencies.

The Fable study factored into its cost and benefit analysis the added construction costs of every evidence-based design innovation, including almost $13 million for larger single-patient rooms, $300,000 for nontoxic building materials and green maintenance protocols, $1 million for the healing garden, $640,000 for "healing art" in public and patient care areas, $374,000 for HEPA filtration systems, $550,000 for water demand reduction, and soon. The total added cost of these features was more than $26 million, which represented a 7.2 percent premium over estimated costs without the features. Because of the study's conservative approach to accounting, that premium was actually somewhat greater than the 0 to 5 percent incremental cost that many of the earliest green hospital construction projects had experienced.

However, the economic value of the improved clinical quality and environmental impacts of the added features, based on evidence from actual hospitals, added up to more than $10 million a year, which resulted in a payback period of just 3 years. Among the significant cost benefits were savings from a 20 percent reduction in hospital-associated infections, a 10 percent reduction in patient length of stay, a 50 percent reduction in

nursing turnover due to increased safety and job satisfaction, an 18 percent reduction in energy demand, and a 30 percent reduction in water
demand, totaling almost 10 million gallons. After the 3-year payback
period, those savings and clinical improvements went straight to Fable's
margin and to the improved health of its patients and staff.

The Fable Hospital's performance on quality and environmental attributes, while only theoretical, was nonetheless confirmed by the experience
of other facilities participating in what was already a rapidly growing trend
in evidence-based hospital design that coincided with the greatest boom
in new hospital construction and renovations in the last half-century.
Between 2000 and 2005, the hospital industry spent nearly $100 billion
in inflation-adjusted dollars on new facilities, up 47 percent from the
previous 5 years, and the red-hot building trend has tilted increasingly
in the direction of evidence-based design, energy efficiency, and environmental mitigation.[18] The trend was driven by a number of converging
forces, including mounting evidence from the Institute of Medicine and
organizations such as the Institute for Healthcare Improvement that documented the shocking number of unnecessary hospital deaths and the solutions available to hospitals for saving millions of patient lives. While much
of the effort focused on improvements in clinical quality and operational
efficiency, the routes to those improvements often involved significant
changes in environmental factors, including alternative energy systems,
improved indoor air quality, substitution of products containing toxic
substances, waste management, and other important green strategies that
have become increasingly commonplace for new and renovated facilities.

DESIGNING HOSPITALS FOR HUMAN AND ENVIRONMENTAL HEALTH

Kaiser Permanente became increasingly involved in promoting the green
hospital movement back in October 2000 when we joined with Health
Care Without Harm as cosponsors of a landmark conference of industry leaders to assess health care's unique environmental opportunities

and challenges. One of the most important outcomes of the Setting Healthcare's Environmental Agenda conference was an agreement that, in the words of architect and evidence-based design champion Gail Vittori, "guidelines and regulations overseeing hospital design and construction should be evaluated based on their impacts on environmental quality and human health and revised so that they reflect these as priority considerations."[19]

About a year after that conference, the American Society of Healthcare Engineering (ASHE) released a "Green Healthcare Construction Guidance Statement," setting out principles for the mitigation of hospitals' environmental impacts that would protect patients, staff, and visitors, as well as surrounding communities and natural resources. In 2002, in response to the need for more specific guidance on our own $24 billion, 26-hospital, 15-year building boom resulting from seismic requirements, we produced our own "Eco-Toolkit" for green facilities, which we shared widely among other pioneering systems.

Our toolkit explicitly stated our aspiration to "limit adverse impacts upon the environment resulting from the siting, design, construction, and operation of our health care facilities," adding that we would "address the life-cycle impacts of facilities through design and construction standards, selection of materials and equipment, and maintenance practices." It also compared the ASHE Guidance Statement approach to the popular US Green Building Council's LEED for New Construction rating system. Although some new hospital projects were registering for LEED certification, most, including Kaiser Permanente, did not. The reason, for us, at least, was that at that time LEED was not designed to meet the unique needs of health care facilities, such as a hospital's unique energy, waste, and indoor air quality requirements. To address these and other green building issues, we developed our own environmental purchasing policy that we continue to use to evaluate the life-cycle environmental impacts of the more than $1 billion worth of products and equipment purchased for all of our 38 hospitals and more than 600 medical offices. It requires architects, engineers, and contractors to specify commercially available and cost-competitive materials, products, and technologies that have a positive impact, or limit negative impacts, on environmental and human health. (See longer discussions of this purchasing policy in Chapters 7 and 8 on health care purchasing and green buildings.) We also advised Health Care Without Harm and the Center for Maximum Potential Building Systems to help create the first of a series of versions of the *Green Guide for Health Care*, a self-rated point system for integrating environmental and health principles and practices into the planning, design, construction, operations, and maintenance of hospitals and other health facilities.

Unlike the LEED certification system, the 360-page *Green Guide for Health Care* did not establish regulatory requirements or minimum standards for design, construction, or operations. It served instead as a voluntary, self-certifying set of metrics and best practices for building green hospitals. Within just a few years, it attracted more than 10,000 registered architects, engineers, and health facilities planners from every state in the nation and 83 other countries. Kaiser Permanente was prominent among them, applying the Green Guide principles to all of our building projects, including our 670,000-square foot Modesto (California) Medical Center, which opened in 2008 as one of the greenest hospitals in the nation at the time.

Looking back, Vittori, co-director of the Center for Maximum Potential Building Systems and one of the prime movers of the green hospital movement, believes the *Green Guide for Health Care* represented a critical turning point in the way new hospitals are conceived and constructed. "In the late 1990s and early 2000s," she recalls, "lots of people in the health care industry said they're in the business of saving lives and weren't focused on environmental issues. But when the *Green Guide for Health Care* came out in 2004, we were finally able to make a strong connection between health and a healthy building, and the green building boom started to gain real momentum."[20]

In the years since, the green building movement in health care has only accelerated, due in part to additional studies attesting to the fact that the physical environment in which patients are treated has a measureable impact on them, as well as on the health of those who care for them.[21] The growing evidence strongly links various design and construction innovations to improved quality and safety outcomes. As Carolyn Clancy, MD, then director of the Agency for Healthcare Research and Quality, noted, "As hospital leaders continue to seek ways to improve quality and reduce errors, it is critical that they look around their own physical environment with the goal of ensuring that the hospital contributes to, rather than impedes, the process of healing."[22]

Also, changes in health care provider reimbursement formulas, such as the Centers for Medicare and Medicaid's recent adoption of pay-for-performance methodologies in Medicare and its new policy of not paying for a variety of preventable patient harms ("never events"), have underscored the overall business case for quality improvement, including the quality and safety of the buildings in which care is provided.

In the latest boost to the green hospital movement, the developers of the *Green Guide for Health Care* collaborated with the US Green Building Council staff to produce a version of the widely used LEED rating system that is unique to the special characteristics of hospitals, including their 24/7 occupancy, patients with compromised immune systems and sensitivities to chemicals and air pollutants, unique regulatory requirements, and the need for fail-safe, efficient energy systems. The new LEED for Healthcare now rates new and renovated health care facilities in five environmental categories, including sustainable siting, water efficiency, energy and atmosphere, materials and resources, and indoor environmental quality. LEED for Healthcare began registering applicants in late 2010, and the full certification system was officially launched the following April. Just 2 years later, in April 2013, the first LEED-Health Care certified medical office building in the nation, Group Health Cooperative's Puyallup Medical Center, opened in Puyallup, Washington, having earned LEED Gold.[23]

While the health care sector has been properly criticized for coming late to the green building movement, it appears to be gaining ground, driven by recent market trends that show a consistent decline in the capital cost premiums for LEED-certified hospital construction, approaching neutrality, over the decade ending in 2012. Studies in 2008 and 2012 showed first-cost premiums of 2.4 percent in 2008 declining to 1.24 percent in 2012, or as low as 0.67 percent for large hospitals (greater than 100,000 square feet).[24] Kaiser Permanente's new hospital near Portland, Oregon, obtained LEED Gold certification for an additional up-front cost of just under $170,000, after Energy Trust of Oregon rebates.

In the most comprehensive study of green building costs and benefits, Greg Kats, an author and former director of financing for energy efficiency and renewable energy at the US Department of Energy, gathered detailed data in 33 states and seven countries on 170 certified-green buildings of all types built between 1998 and 2009. The data were provided directly from the buildings' architects, developers, and owners and included construction costs, energy and water savings, as well as health, productivity, and other green benefits. In *Greening Our Built World*, Kats reports that the vast majority of the green buildings he analyzed had a 0 to 4 percent initial cost premium over similar nongreen buildings, although the greenest buildings, certified as LEED-platinum, had roughly half the cost premium as those with lower certifications, suggesting that quality of the design team is the most important factor in controlling costs of green buildings.[25]

Kats estimates that the average payback period for his data set was 6 years, based on energy savings alone. When water and infrastructure costs, as well as health and employee productivity gains were factored in, the financial benefits more than doubled. And over a 20-year period, the payback exceeded the initial cost premium by four to six times—without including the value to the community of the buildings' reductions in greenhouse gas emissions and other pollutants.

CONCLUSION

Confidence among hospital leaders on the cost-effectiveness of evidence-based design and green construction is clearly nearing a tipping point. In 2011, more than two-thirds (68 percent) of US hospitals that responded to an annual survey by Health Facilities Management and the American Society for Healthcare Engineering (ASHE) claimed to be using environmentally friendly materials in most or all construction and renovation projects, and 60 percent were at least evaluating the costs and benefits of green construction—both percentages up sharply from a year earlier. Also, hospital characteristics that were rare innovations a decade ago, such as use of noise-reducing building materials, improvements in interior air treatment and movement, and efficient, alternative energy systems, are increasingly common in new hospitals, showing up in roughly 30 percent of new facilities."[26]

What will it take to turn the incrementalists driven by the allure of cost savings into full-scale green champions motivated by environmental and human health benefits in addition to bottom-line calculations?

The best hope for turning the green health movement into a standard of business may lie with the 3-year initiative launched in April 2012 by seven leading green health systems, including Advocate Health Care, Dignity Health, Hospital Corporation of America, Inova Health System, Kaiser Permanente, MedStar Health, and Partners HealthCare. Later joined by Bon Secours, Catholic Health Initiatives, Tenet Healthcare, and Vanguard Health Systems, these 11 large systems, with more than $20 billion in annual purchasing power, form the core of the Healthier Hospitals Initiative, discussed in the first chapter. Its aim is to enlist at least 2,000 of the nation's more than 5,000 hospitals over the next few years in dramatically improving the health care sector's environmental footprint, while also saving billions of dollars in costs, and improving the health and safety of millions of patients, staff, and entire communities. In short, HHI is setting out to demonstrate beyond any remaining doubts the triple bottom-line benefits of green health care.

At a White House briefing on the initiative, I represented Kaiser Permanente and was grateful for the opportunity to share some of the highlights of our own green accomplishments in recent years. Surrounded by many of the people I have learned from, collaborated with, and depended on for support and guidance over the last 15 years, it occurred to me during that event that America's health care industry is roughly at the same inflection point I experienced at Kaiser Permanente back in the mid-1990s. Then, as now, a lot of energy and a lot of passion were directed into mostly isolated, grassroots-inspired efforts to promote healthier hospital environments in the interests of healthier patients, staff, communities, and hospital margins. What we needed then to move it to a new level were commitments from our senior leaders, staff coordination of our efforts, strategy, and especially evidence that what we were doing was making a positive difference that was consistent with our mission to provide quality affordable health care. Over the past 15 years, Kaiser Permanente and HHI's other founding health systems, with the help of the key nonprofit advocacy groups, have managed to realize many of our objectives while building, piece by piece, a robust business case for our own green initiatives.

The challenge for health care leaders today is to provide that same mix of leadership, strategy, coordination, and evidence with the objective of transforming not just a single hospital or health system, but the entire US health sector to a deep and healthy shade of green.

NOTES

1. Susan Kaplan, Blair Sadler, Kevin Little, et al., "Can Sustainable Hospitals Help Bend the Health Care Cost Curve?" The Commonwealth Fund, November 2012, http://www.commonwealthfund.org/Publications/Issue-Briefs/2012/Nov/Sustainable-Hospitals.aspx.
2. Healthier Hospitals Initiative, "Study Finds Hospital Environmental Sustainability Efforts Could Save Health Care Sector $15B over 10 Years," press release, November 2, 2012.
3. US EPA, Office of Air Quality Planning & Standards and Office of Research and Development, "Mercury Study Report to Congress: Volume I: Executive Summary," EPA-452/R-97-003, December 1997.
4. John Elkington, "Towards the Sustainable Corporation: Win-Win-Win Business Strategies for Sustainable Development," *California Management Review* 36, no. 2 (1994): 90–100; John Elkington, *Cannibals with Forks: The Triple Bottom Line of 21st Century Business* (Philadelphia: New Society, 1998).
5. Andrew W. Savitz, *The Triple Bottom Line* (San Francisco: John Wiley and Sons, 2006), xiii.
6. US EPA, "Sustainable Materials Management: The Road Ahead, 2020," Executive Summary (June 2009), http://www.epa.gov/epawaste/conserve/smm/pdf/vision2.pdf.
7. Paul Hawken, "Natural Capitalism," *Mother Jones* (March/April 1997), http://www.motherjones.com/politics/1997/03/natural-capitalism.
8. Savitz, *The Triple Bottom Line*, 31.
9. Network for Public Health Law, "Issue Brief: New Requirements for Nonprofit Hospitals Provide Opportunities for Health Department Collaboration" (2011), http://www.networkforphl.org/_asset/fqmqxr/CHNAFINAL.pdf.

10. Kaiser Permanente et al., "Setting Healthcare's Environmental Agenda" (SHEA, 2000).

11. Ray Baxter, interviewed by author and Judith Nemes.

12. Loel Solomon, interviewed by Judith Nemes.

13. Robert Pearl, MD, interviewed by author.

14. Howard Frumkin and Christine Coussen, *Green Healthcare Institutions: Health, Environment, and Economics, Workshop Summary* (Washington, DC: National Academies Press, 2007).

15. B. Millstein, H. Homer, et al., "Why Behavioral and Environmental Interventions Are Needed to Improve Health at Lower Cost," *Health Affairs* 30, no. 5 (May 2011): 1852–1859.

16. John Kouletsis, interviewed by Judith Nemes.

17. Blair L. Sadler et al., "Fable Hospital 2.0: The Business Case for Building Better Health Care Facilities," *Hastings Center Report* 41, no. 1 (2011): 13–23.

18. Dennis Auchon and Julie Appleby, "Hospital Building Booms in 'Burbs," *USA Today*, January 1, 2006.

19. Gail Vittori, "Green and Healthy Buildings for the Healthcare Industry," paper presented at CleanMed conference, Chicago, October 2002.

20. Gail Vitorri, interviewed by Judith Nemes.

21. Anjali Joseph, "The Impact of Light on Outcomes in Healthcare Settings," Center for Health Design Issue Paper no. 2 (2006); Anjali Joseph, "The Impact of the Environment on Infections in Healthcare Facilities," Center for Health Design Issue Paper no. 1 (2006); Anjali Joseph, "The Role of the Physical Environment in Promoting Health, Safety, and Effectiveness in the Healthcare Workplace," The Center for Health Design Issue Paper no. 3 (2006); Anjali Joseph and Roger Ulrich, "Sound Control for Improved Outcomes in Healthcare Settings," Center for Health Design Issue Paper no. 4 (2007).

22. Carolyn Clancy, "Designing for Safety: Evidence-Based Design and Hospitals," *American Journal of Medical Quality* 23, no. 1 (January/February 2008): 68.

23. Elizabeth Powers, "First LEED for Healthcare Certification Complete," US Green Building Council, April 18, 2013, http://www.usgbc.org/articles/first-leed-healthcare-certification-country-complete.

24. Gail Vitorri, "Study: Extra Cost Minimal for LEED-Certified Hospitals," US Green Building Council, October 22, 2013, http://www.usgbc.org/articles/study-extra-costs-minimal-leed-certified-hospitals.

25. Greg Katz, *Greening Our Built World* (Washington, DC: Island Press, 2009).

26. Dave Carpenter, "Hospital Building Report: Shifting Priorities—New Construction Stays Steady While Renovations and Infrasrtucture Get Attention," *Health Facilities Management*, February 2011. http://www.hfmmagazine.com/hfmmagazine/jsp/articledisplay.jsp?dcrpath=HFMMAGAZINE/Article/data/02FEB2011/0211HFM_FEA_CoverStory&domain=HFMMAGAZINE.

4

Food for Health

S troll by Kaiser Permanente's hospital in Oakland, California, on
any Friday morning and you will observe an unlikely scene: doctors, nurses, patients, and others from the surrounding community perusing piles of ripe plums, stacks of fresh corn, and heaps of leafy
greens. Some folks will be chatting with the farmers who come each week
to sell their bounty; others will be tasting slices of fruit or discussing recipes. I stop by this farmers' market whenever I can to pick up fresh organic
produce, but also because I love what it represents. It is a demonstration
that, in addition to treating those who are sick, hospitals can help healthy
people stay that way and avoid the need for their medical care services.
Food at the farmers' market is environmentally beneficial because the
produce is grown using methods that are generally more sustainable than
conventional agriculture, which relies on the intensive use of synthetic
chemicals and fertilizers, is transported much longer distances contributing to carbon dioxide pollution, and results in more packaging waste.

I am especially pleased when I see the familiar face and silver hair of my
recently retired colleague, Preston Maring, MD, who started this market,
picking his way between the cauliflower and strawberries. Dr. Maring
worked for most of his career as a practicing OB-GYN at this hospital. In
2002, he told me, he had an epiphany on a summer day as he was walking through the hospital lobby. He noticed a vendor selling jewelry and

other accessories and thought that selling baubles in a hospital lobby was out of keeping with the values of Kaiser Permanente's medical care program. But the commercial activity made him think of another type of market, one that would fit the organization's focus on prevention and health promotion.

"As a physician, it's clear to me that what people eat has a crucial impact on their health," says Dr. Maring. "The best way to bring people into the fold of eating healthy, locally sourced foods would be to encourage them to cook good food. And what better way to get people started than to host a farmers' market to provide the ingredients?"

Thus was born one of the very first hospital-based farmers' markets in the country—and certainly the first to sell only organic produce. The Oakland market, though small, continues to thrive and has sparked a movement that has spread far and wide. As of 2013, Kaiser Permanente sponsored more than 50 farmers' markets located at our facilities. And thanks in part to Dr. Maring's widely publicized promotion of the concept, the number of farmers' markets sponsored by other hospitals and health systems has come to nearly match the Kaiser Permanente total.[1] So that wonderful scene that unfolds every Friday in Oakland is no longer unique to California or Kaiser Permanente.

In many ways, the farmers' markets are symbolic of a broader movement in health care, closely related to other green health initiatives, to promote healthy and more sustainable food systems. Through their substantial purchasing power and health focus, health care systems are ideally positioned to create change within the wider food system, not only within the hospital walls but throughout the entire food enterprise, from agriculture to food processing, distribution and sales, and preparation and consumption.

Our local hospital farmers' market is just one example of work going on at hospitals and clinics across the country to support local farms and producers, serve healthier, more sustainable offerings to staff and patients, and to make over a tired, industrial food system that until recently served up Jell-O and canned peaches as appropriate hospital food. This work not only seeks to improve health of patients and entire communities but also to improve the well-being of the environment that produces that food.

Examples of health care's growing focus on nutritious, tasty, and sustainably produced food are now cropping up all over the country. Just under 2 hours south of Kaiser Permanente's Oakland hospital, a dedicated team is tending to an expansive garden adjacent to Dominican Hospital in the coastal city of Santa Cruz, California. Sister Mary Ellen Leciejewski, ecology program coordinator for Dominican's umbrella organization, Dignity Health, came up with the idea for the garden in 2003 at about the same time that Dr. Maring was dreaming of farmers' markets at hospitals. By 2009, the garden had grown to 7,350 square feet, and the more than 2,000 pounds of produce grown there each year is served in the hospital's cafeteria. Across the country in Burlington, Vermont, Fletcher Allen Health Care's executive chef is harvesting produce and cooking up gourmet hospital meals from gardens planted on the roof of the hospital's ambulatory care center. The 419-bed hospital buys 80 percent of its beef from local farms that abstain from use of therapeutic antibiotics, and most of the eggs it purchases come from local organic farms.

And at the spectacular Greystone campus of the Culinary Institute of America (CIA) in Napa, California, which trains the nation's top-rated chefs, scores of physicians, dieticians, nurses, other health care professionals, and even hospital administrators come together every spring. They are there to catch up on the latest systematic reviews of nutrition science and to cook up a gastronomic feast of eco-friendly dishes designed to reduce risk of disease and win high marks for patient satisfaction. The 4-day continuing medical education course, sponsored by the CIA and the Harvard School of Public Health, is but one of a growing number of initiatives aimed at reaffirming the importance of healthy, local, and tasty food—how it is produced and processed, purchased, prepared, and served—in the therapeutic regimen of the nation's hospitals.

According to a recent report from the Institute of Medicine, two thirds of adults and almost one third of children in the United States are overweight or obese.[2] This alarming epidemic of excess weight is associated with major causes of chronic disease, disability, and death. Obesity-related illness is estimated to carry an annual cost of $190 billion.[3] And while the ubiquity of high-calorie, fatty, and empty carbohydrate foods is not the only reason for the nation's bulging waistlines, these foods are certainly a major contributor. Since the 1970s, the quantity of food available per person in the United States increased by 16 percent, making far more calories available in the US food supply than are needed.[4]

"We have adopted a dominant food system that, among other features, is producing high-calorie, low-nutrient foods. It does it in a big way in large amounts, and companies are spending billions of dollars a year to market these foods to kids," says Ted Schettler, MD, science director for the Science & Environmental Health Network. "We already have an overwhelming amount of chronic disease. There's a place for a much stronger voice in this area from the health care system."[5]

Current epidemics of chronic disease are not the only price we pay for the remarkable efficiency of the nation's food system. Its large-scale model of production and distribution has also contributed to unprecedented levels of environmental damage: industrial pollution of air and water, creation and spread of antibiotic-resistant bacteria, the spread of food-borne pathogens, climate-changing emissions related to food transportation and processing, and contamination of agricultural lands and water tables from chemicals and pesticides.

A few important examples of our industrial food system's environmental impacts:

- About 30 percent of global emissions that lead to climate change are attributable to agricultural activities, including land use changes such as deforestation.
- The US food system accounts for an estimated 19 percent of the nation's consumption of greenhouse gas–emitting fossil fuels.
- Experts agree that antibiotic use in agriculture contributes to rising drug-resistant infections in humans. An estimated 80 percent of all antibiotics consumed in the United States are used as nontherapeutic feed additives for poultry, swine, and beef cattle to promote growth and to compensate for diseases caused by poor animal husbandry.[6]

Clearly, it will take more than farmers' markets, hospital gardens, and sustainable food conferences to make a dent in the nation's predominant system of food production. Where the health care sector can really make a difference is by flexing the muscle inherent in the $12 billion per year it spends annually on food.[7]

Many hospitals and health systems are already using their purchasing power to promote sustainable agriculture practices and a healthier food system. More than 400 hospitals have signed the Healthy Food in Health Care Pledge, created by Health Care Without Harm, which means they are committing to buying locally sourced food, reducing the amount of food they serve that contains pesticides, growth hormones, or antibiotics, and adopting sustainable food procurement policies. In some cases, they are also using their influence to change public policy on topics ranging from the availability of sugar-sweetened beverages to antibiotics in food production and reform of federal laws governing agriculture. And in hundreds of hospitals across the country, food service managers are finding ways to tap into sustainable, regional food systems. And local, seasonal fruit is turning up on patient trays, meat entrees free of growth hormones and antibiotics are being offered in employee cafeterias, and fair trade coffee and healthier snacks are showing up in hospital vending machines.

EMERGING FROM THE INDUSTRIAL PARADIGM

Food issues—ranging from farm policy to pesticide use, antibiotics, and the question of genetically modified organism (GMO) labeling—are now in the news on an almost daily basis. But for a long time in the post–World War II era, food in the United States was almost invisible as a political or health care issue. Cheap fossil fuel (the key ingredient in both chemical fertilizers and pesticides) and changes to agriculture policy in the 1970s pushed food prices lower, especially for processed foods made from highly subsidized crops like corn and soy, as opposed to fresh fruits and vegetables, which became ever more expensive.[8] The result was a bountiful harvest of inexpensive, packaged foods that now oversupplies

Americans with about 3,900 calories per person per day, far above the 2,000–2,500 calorie recommendation.[9] And those calories are not only more plentiful but also much cheaper, presenting consumers with food choices that, in terms of price, completely contradict the US Department of Agriculture's (USDA) dietary recommendations. Americans now spend as little as 6.6 percent of their income on food eaten at home, or about half as much as most Europeans spend.[10]

Concerns over the health impacts of the industrial food system came to light in the early 1970s and 1980s with a series of food safety scandals, including mad cow disease, which focused attention on the way that food was being produced. Following a wave of food-borne poisonings involving tainted eggs, peanut butter, and spinach in 2010, Congress passed the Food Safety and Modernization Act, creating greater government oversight of food production and processing. But 3 years later the *New York Times* cited government estimates that one in six Americans were still falling ill from contaminated food products every year, resulting in 130,000 annual hospitalizations and 3,000 deaths.[11]

Clearly, new technologies in agriculture and food processing have helped to create a vast supply of cheap food, which undeniably has had some beneficial impacts on Americans' standard of living. But the growing number of serious food-related health scares indicates that those benefits have come at a high price—a price often paid in a growing and ever-more costly list of acute and chronic health conditions for both the planet and its people.

HEALTH CARE JOINS THE MOVEMENT

Health care organizations, including the early pioneers of the green health movement, were slow to catch on to the double-edged nature of the industrial food revolution. As was the case for toxics and harmful chemicals in health care, it took a self-taught idealist from a non–health care background to help wake people up to health care's responsibilities in modeling and promoting healthy, environmentally sustainable food policies (see Box 4.1).

Box 4.1   WHAT IS "SUSTAINABLE"?

A good reference for defining sustainable food is the *Green Guide for Health Care*'s Food Service Credits (http://www.gghc.org/resources.greenoperations.food.php). The *Green Guide for Health Care*'s credit system is a benchmarking tool, developed by Health Care Without Harm and the Center for Maximum Potential Building Systems, specifically for sustainable food in health care. Some examples of how Kaiser Permanente applies this criteria include food produced within 250 miles of where it is served; food produced without pesticides, antibiotics, or added hormones; and food certified as sustainably produced by a third-party eco-label. Food products must meet at least one of these criteria to be considered sustainable, though preference is given to products that meet multiple criteria. Using this definition, Kaiser Permanente devotes about 18 percent of its overall food spending to sustainably produced food across the organization. Kaiser Permanente intends to grow that to 20 percent by the end of 2015.

For many in health care, the person who first raised the alarms about unhealthy food policies in health care was Jamie Harvie, a civil engineer who was active in the early prevention efforts around toxic pollution and the national mercury elimination campaign. Harvie called me in 2004, at a time when he was working on a range of issues at the intersection of public health and ecological health, including development of sustainable food policies. He floated the idea of bringing together a group of clinicians, nongovernmental organizations, and health care institutions to discuss how we could better act on the important connections between patient health, community health, environmental health, and the food purchased and served by health care facilities.

Less than a year later, in November, 2005, Harvie persuaded 200 people to come together just a few blocks from Kaiser Permanente's Oakland headquarters in what would be the first annual conference known as FoodMed. Encouraged by the response from participants, he went on to help start the

Healthy Food in Health Care program, a national initiative of Health Care Without Harm, to demonstrate that, in his words, "by purchasing foods that are produced, processed, and transported in ways that protect public and environmental health, hospitals can make a profound difference in the market and in the food settings of the people they serve."[12]

The following year, Healthy Food in Health Care launched its Healthy Food Pledge so that hospitals and health systems could send a message to the marketplace about their commitment to "local, nutritious, and sustainable food." The more than 430 hospitals that have since signed the pledge commit to the following:

- Increase their offerings of fruit, vegetables, and minimally processed, unrefined foods.
- Reduce unhealthful trans- and saturated fats and sweetened foods.
- Procure for their cafeterias readily obtainable, socially responsible, and sustainable foods like milk from cows that have not been given bovine growth hormone, fair trade coffee, and, where possible, organic produce.
- Work with local farmers, community-based organizations, and food suppliers to increase the availability of fresh, locally produced food.
- Encourage their suppliers to offer food that is grown or raised in identifiable systems that eliminate the use of toxic pesticides, hormones, and nontherapeutic antibiotics—systems that support farmer and farm worker health and welfare.
- Educate their patients and community about the nutritious, socially just, and ecologically sustainable healthy food practices they have embraced.
- Minimize and beneficially reuse food waste.
- Report annually on their progress in meeting these goals.

More recently, Healthy Food in Health Care and other organizations, including Kaiser Permanente and other health systems, have come together to form the Healthier Hospitals Initiative (described previously), which asks member hospitals and health systems to commit to a series of challenges in six related areas. The food challenges include the following:

- Adopting a sustainable food policy for the organization.
- Decreasing the amount of meat purchased by 20 percent within 3 years.
- Increasing the percentage of healthy beverage purchases by 20 percent of total beverage purchases annually, or achieving healthy beverage purchases of 80 percent of total beverage purchases for use throughout the hospital within 3 years.
- Increasing the percentage of local and/or sustainable food purchases by 20 percent annually, or achieving local and/or sustainable food purchases of 15 percent of total food dollar purchases within 3 years.

HEALTH IMPLICATIONS: WHY SUSTAINABLE FOOD IS A HEALTH CARE ISSUE

Overweight and Obesity

"Let food be thy medicine and medicine be thy food," said Hippocrates. But presumably, the father of Western medicine did not have in mind the nutritiously challenged processed foods that today make up about 70 percent of the average American's diet.[13] Nor was he thinking of a population, such as ours, in which generous servings of pesticide- and chemical-free fruits and vegetables had almost disappeared from the average meal. And he certainly was not contemplating a time when the average adult would spend a mere half-hour a day engaged in preparing meals and cleaning up after them, thanks to readily available fast foods from drive-through restaurants and other such conveniences.[14]

Clearly, the food we eat and decreased physical activity are contributing to a wide array of costly and debilitating health problems, beginning with the epidemic of overweight and obesity, which affects two thirds of adults and almost one third of children in the United States. As mentioned previously, the estimated annual medical cost of obesity in this country is $190 billion, and the cost of human suffering is even greater. Obese children are more likely to have high blood pressure and high cholesterol, which are important risk factors for many of the nation's leading causes of preventable death, including cardiovascular disease, stroke, type 2 diabetes, and certain types of cancer. Obesity is also a risk factor for breathing problems like sleep apnea and asthma, joint problems and musculoskeletal disorders, fatty liver disease, gallstones, and social and psychological problems, including cognitive impairment, dementia, and Alzheimer's disease.[15]

Chemical Contamination of Food from Pesticides and Fertilizers

After the publication of Rachel Carson's book *Silent Spring* 50 years ago, the dangers of pesticide use came into sharper focus, resulting in the banning of some pesticides and improvements for wildlife and human health. Now, however, American agriculture is using more pesticides than ever.

About 1.2 billion pounds of pesticides are used in the United States annually,[16] and they are responsible for a broad array of negative health effects. Although farm workers and their families and residents who live in areas near pesticide-treated fields are most at risk, everyone who consumes foods with pesticide residues also carries pesticides and their by-products in his or her body. Exposure to pesticides also results from contaminated air, water, and soil far from the treated fields, which together with contaminated foods account for the fact that a wide range of pesticide-related chemicals are now detectable in the blood of most pregnant women in the United States.[17] Like other environmental chemicals, food-related chemicals can enter the fetus of pregnant women and cause birth defects, preterm birth, low birth weight, childhood cancers, congenital anomalies, neurobehavioral and cognitive deficits, and asthma.[18] There is also mounting evidence of a connection between early exposure to certain pesticides and Parkinson's disease, a degenerative disorder of the central nervous system. "To a disturbing extent," concluded the annual President's Cancer Panel Report in 2010, "babies are born 'prepolluted.'"[19]

A 2009 study of the cumulative pesticide burden in children estimated that 40 percent of US children have enough exposure to pesticides to potentially impact their brains and nervous systems.[20] For many of these children, food is probably the key pathway for pesticide exposure, as illustrated by a study that found drastic, immediate reductions of pesticide metabolites in children who were placed on an organic, pesticide-free diet.[21]

Researchers are "concerned about shedding more light on pesticides in the food system because it's all integrated, and food is a key driver to reproductive health," says Patrice Sutton, a research scientist in the Program on Reproductive Health and the Environment at the University of San Francisco and lead author of an influential 2011 review of research on the reproductive health consequences of pesticides and other food-related chemicals.[22] "We're not just talking about concerns over good birth outcomes. We're talking about health across the lifespan of the individual and potentially the impact across multiple generations. Many of these chronic diseases later in life, such as diabetes and cardiovascular disease, also are extremely costly."

Pesticides are not the only health concern in modern industrialized agriculture. Since the so-called Green Revolution of the 1960s that saw the development of very high-yield crops, inorganic, chemical fertilizers have largely replaced organic fertilizers, and the use of these has reached staggering proportions. In 2013, worldwide demand reached a new record of 182 million tons, up from 168 million tons in 2007, and new records are set every year.[23] These fertilizers contain nitrogen, phosphorus, and/or potassium, and they are manufactured through an energy-intensive process that requires the burning of fossil fuels. Additionally, nitrogen-based fertilizers, which account for the great majority of all chemical fertilizers, can leech nitrates into sources of drinking water, which has been linked to "blue baby syndrome" (methemoglobiemia) and higher risks of reproductive health impacts and cancer.[24]

Food on Steroids

If Hippocrates were to visit a modern American concentrated animal feedlot operation (CAFO), he might reconsider his statement equating food with medicine. Over the last several decades, the industrial food system has adopted the widespread practice of intentionally giving natural and synthetic steroid hormones, antibiotics, and even arsenic to beef cattle, poultry, and other livestock. The practice is not intended to treat sick animals but to encourage them to grow larger, faster, and to prevent them from spreading infections as a result of living in large, crowded, confined CAFOs and similar quarters. These additives are being passed along to humans via our hamburgers, chicken wings, and other meat and poultry products, as well as through contaminated water tables. In humans, these residues in our food and water are just the opposite of medicinal, posing potential risks to natural hormone function, reproductive health, and other physiological functions.[25] Scientific evidence of those risks has been sufficient for many other industrialized countries, including the European Union, to restrict or prohibit giving these additives to healthy food animals. But the practice remains legal and widespread in the United States, despite ongoing legislative efforts to impose restrictions.

The use of antibiotics in cattle and other food animals is of particular concern to public health authorities. Antibiotics are an invaluable resource for treating infections in humans, and they are among the most common drugs in medicine. But the overuse of antibiotics and antimicrobials in both humans and animals has resulted in alarmingly high levels of resistant strains of bacteria and other pathogens. According to a 2013 report by the US Centers for Disease Control and Prevention (CDC), at least 2 million Americans acquire serious illnesses from pathogens that are resistant to one or more of the antibiotics designed to treat those conditions—including the bacteria that cause tuberculosis, the viruses that cause influenza, the parasites that cause malaria, and the fungi that cause yeast infections. This is incurring an estimated cost of $20 billion in excess direct health care cost, with additional social costs as high as $35 billion a year. "At least 23,000 people die each year as a direct result of these antibiotic-resistant infections," states the report, and "many more die from other conditions that were complicated by an antibiotic-resistant infection."[26] It notes that recently evolved superbugs, like MRSA (methicillin-resistant staph aureus) strike at least 80,000 patients a year, and more than 11,000 result in death.

Dr. Tom Frieden, director of the CDC, called the rising rate of antibiotic resistance "an urgent health threat," adding, "We talk about a pre-antibiotic era and an antibiotic era. If we're not careful, we will soon be in a post-antibiotic era. The medicine chest will be empty when we go there, to look for a life-saving antibiotic."

Physicians who are faced with the problem of antibiotic resistance firsthand are at the head of the queue for those working to restrict nontherapeutic antibiotics in animal feed. Dr. Thomas Newman, a pediatrician at the University of California, San Francisco (UCSF) Medical Center who has been involved in a variety of environmental efforts on behalf of Physicians for Social Responsibility, is one of them. "I get angry because here I am worrying about prescribing antibiotics for ear infections, and I hear they are mixing it into animal food," he says. "I think it's time for health care organizations to say we're just not going to buy this stuff anymore. There's no excuse for it. It's harmful to human and animal health."[27] In May 2013, Newman spearheaded the approval of a resolution by UCSF's academic senate to phase out meat raised with nontherapeutic antibiotics in the medical center's food service.[28]

However, finding solutions can be vexing. Hospital food purchasers nationwide are having difficulty finding chickens that have not been given antibiotics, arsenic, or other additives in sufficient quantity and at a reasonable cost to replace conventional supply (see Box 4.2). At Kaiser Permanente, for instance, Jan Villarante, director of National Nutrition Services, says it has been difficult to find a good supply of antibiotic-free chickens that her staff would not have to pluck themselves. But, despite the challenge of having to source some 72,800 chickens a year for patient meals, Villarante and her staff have been able to start purchasing chicken raised without antibiotics. She estimates that starting in 2014 Kaiser

Permanente will be purchasing more than 100,000 pounds of this sustainable chicken annually, and plans are under way to purchase beef raised without antibiotics. "We know the farmers out there who want to help us," she says, "and now we're working on the regional processing plants to get the product we want."

Box 4.2   FLETCHER ALLEN TAKES ON "DRUGGED" FOODS

When the food procurement managers at Fletcher Allen Health Care in Burlington, Vermont, signed the Healthy Food Pledge in 2006, its first priority was to reduce antibiotics and hormones in the food supply for the 550-bed hospital, recalls Diane Imrie, director of nutrition services. The hospital, which serves 2 million meals a year to its patients and employees, embarked on an ambitious 3-year plan to stop buying beef, poultry, pork, fish, cheese, and eggs that contained any hormones or antibiotics.

"I was seeing an increasing number of patients with multiple antibiotic-resistant infections and the numbers were rampant across the country," explains Imrie. "It's one of those things that's indicative of a bad food system, and I was passionate about getting antibiotics out of our hospital food. We may not impact our patients' health with that change in menu because they're only here two or three days. But some of our employees work here for forty years and eat two meals a day here."

By 2010, Imrie and her colleagues had achieved most of their goal. That year, they were able to purchase all antibiotic-free items in just about every category, and as much as 90 percent of their beef supply. Pot roast was the lone holdout where no substitute could be found, laments Imrie. Pork was a challenge, too, for a while. Her solution: "We took all pork off the menu for a few years because we couldn't find anything on the market that was without antibiotics at a price we could afford."

Chemically Treated Food Packaging

In addition to the chemicals of concern that are found in or on the products of industrialized farming, there also is reason to worry about the
chemicals used in food packaging.

STYRENE

Styrene, which can leach from polystyrene (Styrofoam) cups, plates, and
carry-out containers when heated, has been shown to be potentially toxic
to humans as a neurotoxin and carcinogen.[29] Animal studies have demonstrated that styrene also can have an adverse effect on red blood cells, the
liver, kidneys, and the stomach.

BISPHENOL-A

Bisphenol-A, or BPA, is a chemical present in a wide array of food and
drink containers. It has been banned from use in baby bottles and drinking cups for children in some states, but it is still found as a liner in many
baby food containers and other products for the general population. It is
also in some water bottles, plastic dinnerware, and clear plastic cutlery.

Hundreds of studies in animals, and more recently some studies in
humans, have documented myriad health problems related to BPA exposure.
It is a known disruptor of hormones in the human body. Links have been
found with early-life exposure to BPA and reproductive and developmental
problems, as well as cancer and diabetes. Studies have shown BPA exposure
can cause genetic damage, which can lead to miscarriages and birth defects.[30]

PHTHALATES

Phthalates represent a group of chemicals that are found in some plastic food
packaging, as well as other consumer products. They are known hormone
disruptors and can leach into oily or fatty foods when they come into con-
tact or when they are heated. Health problems include adverse effects on the
liver, kidney, spleen, bone formation, and body weight.[31] In addition, there is
concern they may be cancer-causing agents. Researchers have found connections between phthalate exposure and liver and thyroid toxicity, reproductive
abnormalities, and problems with the respiratory system, such as asthma.

THE FOOD SYSTEM'S IMPACT ON CLIMATE CHANGE

If the world's dominant food production/distribution system of the past half century has posed major challenges to human health, it has been no less problematic for the health of the environment. According to a detailed 2012 report by the Consultive Group on International Agricultural Research (CGIAR), the industrialized, chemical, and transport-dependent food system accounts for about a third of all greenhouse gas emissions through land use change and direct emissions.[32] Agricultural production is responsible for the lion's share of those emissions, followed by fertilizer manufacture, refrigeration, transport, and indirect emissions from deforestation and land-use changes. The report found that the overall global food system released the equivalent of 9,800–16,900 megatons of carbon dioxide into the atmosphere in 2008. A separate study, by the UN Food and Agriculture Organization, estimates that livestock production alone is responsible for 18 percent of all human-caused greenhouse gases, due mainly to the use of fossil fuels to boost grain production to feed livestock.[33]

POLICY REFORMS FOR A HEALTHIER FOOD SYSTEM

Reforming the existing global and US food system to prioritize human and environmental health and safety will require the engagement of all sectors of society, public and private, local and global. On the public policy front, much of the action will involve the United Nations and other global food, agriculture, and trade organizations, given that the US food system is a global system involving massive food exports and imports with more than 150 countries through more than 300 ports of entry.

Many public health, environmental, and health professional groups have been involved in efforts to reform the major federal laws governing US food production and safety, focusing primarily on the Farm Bill, which is reauthorized every 5 years and includes hundreds of programs that influence the food production and distribution systems. It is the primary agricultural and food policy tool of the federal government and addresses issues such as nutrition, food stamps, conservation programs, agriculture, trade, and more. Advocates of sustainable food and agriculture policies have largely focused on reforms that accomplish the following objectives:

- Support new and existing small and mid-sized farms capable of competing for local markets with industrialized megafarms.
- Support creation of local and regional food systems that are not dependent on transporting foods over thousands of miles from farm to market, thus reducing air pollution and its associated greenhouse gases and respiratory illnesses.
- Strengthen the authority and resources of the US FDA to protect the food supply through better routine monitoring, screening, and enforcement activities.
- Promote a shift of federal farm subsidies from corn, wheat, and soybeans to "green subsidies," including healthier fruits and vegetables.
- Promote more sustainable farming methods that protect human and environmental health, including restricted use of synthetic pesticides, growth hormones, nontherapeutic antibiotics, and CAFOs.[34]

CASE STUDIES: HOW HEALTH CARE ORGANIZATIONS ARE CREATING HEALTHY FOOD SOLUTIONS FOR PEOPLE AND THE PLANET

It is easy to become overwhelmed with the daunting array of health issues surrounding food in health care. But in a relatively short time, the broader green health movement has spawned hundreds, or even thousands, of creative pilot programs and ambitious, well-researched, full-bore food policies aimed at putting human and environmental health at the center of every patient food tray, employee cafeteria, and vending machine. Scores of hospitals and large health systems are also reaching out to their surrounding communities to effect positive changes in the local food and agriculture environment through community benefit activities. In towns and cities across the nation, hospitals are doing the following:

- Purchasing and serving less meat and dairy.
- Substituting sustainably produced meat and dairy products and nutritionally balanced vegetarian options.
- Serving grass-fed, certified organic and other foods produced without use of fossil fuel–based fertilizers and pesticides.
- Eliminating use of bottled water.
- Reducing, reusing, or composting food waste, among many other activities.

Progress at Kaiser Permanente

Kaiser Permanente has taken a measured approach that reflects how progress is possible, even within such a large institution. With 38 hospitals, the organization serves 14,000 patient meals each day. Although the large scale poses serious challenges, it is also an advantage in that it allows Kaiser Permanente to influence the market with purchasing power.

A movement that started with the idea for one farmers' market years ago has now grown to include a wide array of activities and accomplishments, including the following:

- About 590 tons of the fruits and vegetables served on patient menus (nearly 50 percent of all fresh produce that Kaiser Permanente purchases) are sustainably and/or locally produced.
- About 6 percent of fruits and vegetables purchased are certified organic, about double the level of overall consumption of organic produce in the United States.
- Kaiser Permanente now hosts or sponsors more than 50 farmers' markets at our hospitals and medical centers across the country.
- All coffee and tea in Kaiser Permanente vending machines is fair trade.

- As of January 1, 2014, 18 percent of Kaiser Permanente's total
  food spending is on sustainable food, and the goal is to achieve
  20 percent by year-end 2015.
- All milk and yogurt served with patient meals and in cafeterias
  and vending machines is free of the growth hormone rBGH.
- Kaiser Permanente now serves cage-free Certified Humane
  Raised and Handled eggs on its Northern California patient
  menu.
- In April 2012, Kaiser Permanente began serving burgers made
  with beef that is free of antibiotics and added hormones on its
  Northern California patient menu.
- Kaiser Permanente's Southern California Region eliminated
  sweetened beverages in vending machines, cafeterias, and
  medical centers and has removed deep fat fryers. Other Kaiser
  Permanente regions are following suit.
- Kaiser Permanente has reduced beef purchases by 18 percent
  through plant-based menu options.
- In October 2012, Kaiser Permanente signed onto Partnership for
  a Healthier America in support of Michelle Obama's Let's Move
  Program. It includes goals for increasing the amount of fruits
  and vegetables offered and promoting healthy food options.
- Kaiser Permanente provides major funding and technical assistance
  through Community Benefit activities for local and national
  nonprofits promoting sustainable food and agriculture practices.

Sustainable Food Purchasing

When we were looking for new contractors and distributors for our
food purchasing, we were able to introduce an innovative scorecard tool
to evaluate the environmental sustainability of each potential vendor
based on the information they were required to provide to us as part of
the bid process. The "Sustainable Food Scorecard," based in part on our
Sustainability Scorecard for Medical Purchasing (see Chapter 7), requires

potential vendors to provide details regarding their corporate and distribution practices.

Kaiser Permanente used this information to compare competing vendors' commitments to sustainability, as well as their ability to identify sustainable products in their order guides, and to track and report on our overall spending on sustainable food. The scorecard also required vendors to provide detailed lists of sustainable food and nonfood offerings, and how each line item met Kaiser Permanente's Sustainable Food Purchasing Criteria. Vendor responses to the scorecard were a key factor in selecting our current contractor and distributor. We have shared the Sustainable Food Scorecard through Practice Greenhealth to help establish sustainable food standards for the entire industry.

FOOD HUBS AND COOPERATIVES

Food hubs and cooperatives are another format for bringing together hospitals looking for local food with the producers who can give them what they want.

In Wisconsin, Gundersen Lutheran health system played a pivotal role as an anchor and founding member of a regional food cooperative that brings local, sustainable smaller farmers and food producers together to aggregate their goods and efficiently connect them to participating buyers nearby. The 325-bed hospital, located in La Crosse, helped establish the Fifth Season Cooperative in 2010 with a handful of other partners that wanted to buy healthy food in the region and support the local economy, says Tom J. Thompson, the hospital's sustainability coordinator.[35]

"We're famous in Wisconsin for our cheese, but there's lots of delicious meat and produce here too," shares Thompson, who notes the hospital made a commitment to buy 20 percent of its food from local sources. "It makes no sense to go further away to buy great food that's right here at our doorstep."

In 2011, some items the hospital was buying through the cooperative included sustainably grown summer and fall produce, and all-beef hot dogs made from local, grass-fed, hormone-free, and antibiotic-free cattle.

Other participants in the co-op include the University of Wisconsin-La Crosse, the Viroqua Area School District, CROPP (an organic farmers' cooperative with its well-known Organic Valley brand), Premier Meats, and Willow Creek Ranch. The hospital convinced its larger distributor to join the co-op as a way of increasing the local options it can provide to customers (including Gundersen Lutheran) and providing more buying power to strengthen the future viability of Fifth Season.

In a different configuration, distribution centers are popping up around the country to help connect the dots that get local farmers into the distribution system so hospitals, schools, restaurants, and other institutional buyers can get access to their goods. Puget Sound Food Network, based in Mount Vernon, Washington, has developed a successful model in the Pacific Northwest and gets calls from hospitals around the country for advice on how to solve access and distribution problems in their markets.

In Michigan, the state Health and Hospitals Association adopted an innovative four-star program that encourages member hospitals to buy local, sustainable foods within the state's boundaries and serve healthier food as part of a larger campaign to reduce obesity rates and promote wellness. In 2010, the trade association asked its 137 hospital members to sign a pledge promising, in part, to shift at least 20 percent of their food procurement to Michigan producers and processors by 2020, says Brian Peters, the group's executive vice president of operations. The response was overwhelming. By late 2011, 86 hospitals had signed the pledge and some were already buying more than 20 percent of their foods from local sources.

"We have one of the highest obesity rates in the country and Michigan's new governor at the time identified obesity as a significant issue," recalls Peters. "We saw that the old model of paying hospitals for volume was going away and we saw an incentive to engage in population management by encouraging people to be healthy. As hospitals, we need to lead by setting a good example. If we can't get rid of industrial trans fats in our hospitals, we can't ask restaurants and others to do it, either."

Hospitals can be an ideal drop-off point for community-supported agriculture, or CSA, programs, which help support local farmers and offer healthy produce for hospital staff, patients, and participating community members. A CSA program essentially is a partnership between a local farm and a group of members who choose to support the producer by paying for food upfront as a "share" in the CSA and then receiving deliveries of fresh goods during the harvesting season. The farm gets a guaranteed investment at the beginning of the season, which enables owners to do long-term planning for their own viability and strengthens the sometimes unstable nature of local food systems.

Many hospitals nationwide are already partnering with nearby growers and establishing CSAs at their facilities. They include Boston Medical Center; Children's Hospital of Philadelphia; Baystate Franklin Medical Center in Greenfield, Massachusetts; and Legacy Health in Portland, Oregon. The popularity of these programs is expected to increase as more good stories are shared and as more hospitals reach out to find CSAs in their region.

Another example of group purchasing from local producers is taking root right in the San Francisco Bay Area. A group of local hospitals, including the UCSF Medical Center, John Muir Health, the San Francisco VA Medical Center, San Francisco General Hospital, and Kaiser Permanente are pooling their purchasing of locally grown produce to bring more of the fresh fruits and vegetables onto patient plates and into employee cafeterias. Kaiser Permanente's Dr. Maring, who started the farmers' markets, played a leading role in this project, as are San Francisco Bay Area Physicians for Social Responsibility and the Community Alliance with Family Farmers. The effort, known as the Regional Produce Purchasing Project, aims to support local farmers by creating a steady demand from the health care sector. It also means a lot more locally grown produce is making its way into hospitals.

The concept is spreading to Southern California and potentially to other parts of the country. "When we started our first farmers' market, we were focused on one hospital in one community," says Dr. Maring. "Now, we realize that the more we can collaborate, the better chance we have to help create a healthier food system and healthier people."

Moving Forward with the Healthier Hospitals Initiative

Clearly, progress is being made by health systems throughout the country. The key to moving to an even greater level of achievement, I believe, lies in the ability to move together, in collaboration. Looking ahead, I am convinced that future progress in the sustainable food area will come as hospitals and health systems pool their purchasing power and use their credibility and community leadership to articulate and spread a vision of sustainable, healthy food throughout US society. An example of such collaboration discussed earlier is the Healthier Hospitals Initiative (HHI) food challenge. Following are a few case studies from the many examples of inspiring work by current HHI members to put health at the heart of their food policies.

CASE STUDIES OF HEALTHY FOOD INITIATIVES IN HEALTH CARE

Less Meat, More Veggies: The Balanced Menus Challenge

Health Care Without Harm teamed up with the HHI to sponsor the Balanced Menus Challenge to encourage hospitals to reduce their meat and poultry purchases by 20 percent and invest their cost savings in sustainable meat options. The sponsors claim that Americans eat more than twice the global average for meat consumption, or nearly 9 ounces of meat and chicken per day, in contrast to the USDA recommendation of 5.5 ounces per day. Many hospital food service operations mirror this overconsumption, serving meat with one to two meals per day. Reducing the overall amount of meat served in hospitals provides important health, social, and environmental benefits that are consistent with prevention-based medicine.

Metro West Medical Center in Framingham, Massachusetts, took the Balanced Menus challenge by the relatively simple step of incorporating "Meatless Mondays" into the hospital's cafeteria menu, says Addie Gibson, operations manager for support services.[36] They also found smaller ways to tweak the menu and take meat ingredients out of recipes whenever possible. Just about all the soups there are now vegetable based, and they are serving more pasta primavera and omitting the meat sauces, Gibson says. The hospital also eliminated all meats from the patient breakfast menu, but it will give it to patients if they ask for it.

The food program at the San Francisco VA Hospital met the challenge by redesigning its patient menu to feature a doubling of vegetable portions and salads and reducing meat portions to 2–3 ounces. It also set up a local sourcing program for fresh fruits, vegetables, and nuts. At nearby UCSF Medical Center, food service leaders reduced its beef menu items from 42 to 3, cut beef purchases by 36 percent in 9 months, and ensured that 10 of its 14 soup offerings would be vegetarian.[37]

In Portland, Oregon, Oregon Health and Science's Food and Nutrition Services began working with local ranchers in 2010 to establish a so-called farm-to-fork program. The medical center now offers Food Alliance–certified, grass-fed, finished beef with no added hormones or antibiotics. OHSU purchases four to five cows each week, using the bones for house-made soup stocks and major cuts for the retail menu. The rest of the meat is ground and either prepared for burgers and meatloaf for patient and retail menus or packed away in the freezer for winter. The pasture-fed beef from the main supplier, Carmen Ranch, is lower in calories, saturated fat, and cholesterol than conventionally raised beef.[38]

Eliminating Sugar-Sweetened Beverages

The HHI food challenge includes increasing the percentage of healthy beverage purchases by 20 percent annually over the baseline year or achieving healthy beverage purchases of 80 percent of total beverage purchases for use throughout the hospital. The most direct way to do this is the elimination of all sugar-sweetened beverages (SSBs), as some of the health systems noted earlier have done. This is precisely what St. Elizabeth Medical Center, a part of Steward Health Care System in Boston, did.

An SSB is defined as any beverage with an added caloric sweetener (sugar or other). A typical 20-ounce soda can contain 16 teaspoons of sugar and 250 calories. Besides having vital health benefits, the elimination of SSBs has real environmental benefits, since the industrial systems that make high-fructose corn syrup and similar sweeteners cheap and plentiful rely on fossil fuel–based chemicals and toxic pesticides.

St. Elizabeth's Medical Center, a 272-bed hospital affiliated with Tufts University School of Medicine, kicked off its healthy beverage program in 2011 by eliminating more than 20 varieties of SSBs from coolers and drink fountains. Product placement of healthier options, paired with a shift in pricing structure, were part of the strategy. In addition to replacing soda advertisements on vending machines, a color-coded beverage system was added, featuring red, yellow, and green signage to help make buying the right thing the easy thing. Also, filtered water machines were added in the main cafeteria to promote free drinking water. The results were impressive: a 49 percent reduction in SSB cafeteria purchases. The focus will now turn to elimination of SSBs from patient menus.[39]

The Dartmouth-Hitchcock Medical Center in Lebanon, New Hampshire, has taken a similar step by banning SSB sales in dining areas, vending machines, and the food court's commercial vendors, like Au Bon Pain and Sbarro. SSBs were targeted because they are the quintessential empty-calorie food, high in calories and low in nutrition, said hospital spokesman Rick Adams. "Decreasing the calories from beverages can lead to greater weight reduction than reducing calories in solid food," he noted, adding that "There's some pretty strong evidence that sugar-sweetened beverages are linked to various illnesses," including obesity, diabetes, and heart disease. According to a survey in 2010, six in ten medical center employees were overweight. Presumably, many of them were among the workers, patients, and visitors who shed an estimated 1,400 pounds of body weight in the first year of the ban.[40]

Similarly impressive results were achieved by Huron Valley Sinai Hospital in Commerce, Michigan, where 2 months after transitioning to healthier beverages, sales of sugar-sweetened drinks fell by nearly $7,000 while sales of healthier beverages rose by nearly $8,000. Based on a 20-ounze bottle of Coke as an "average" container, the facility estimates it removed more than 1 million pounds of sugar from its cafeteria in 2 months.

NOTES

1. David Ollier Weber, "A Simple Recipe for Community Benefit," *H&HN Daily*, February 26, 2013, http://www.hhnmag.com/hhnmag/HHNDaily/HHNDaily Display.dhtml?id =2510003767.
2. National Research Council. *Accelerating Progress in Obesity Prevention: Solving the Weight of the Nation* (Washington, DC: National Academies Press, 2012).
3. J. Cawley and C. Meyerhoefer, "The Medical Care Costs of Obesity: An Instrumental Variables Approach," *Journal of Health Economics* 31, no. 1 (2012): 219–230.
4. H. Farah and J. C. Buzby, "US Food Consumption up 16 Percent Since 1970," *Amber Waves* (November 2005), http://www.ers.usda.gov/AmberWaves/November05/findings/usfoodconsumption.htm; US Department of Agriculture Economic Research Service, "Food Availability (Per Capita) Data System: Data Sets 2011," http://www.ers.usda.gov/Data/FoodConsumption/ (accessed March 10, 2012).
5. Ted Schettler, interviewed by the author.
6. Kaiser Permanente Institute for Health Policy, "Supporting Individual and Environmental Health Through Sustainable Food Procurement," *Kaiser Permanente Policy Story* 1, no. 7 (2012), http://www.kpihp.org/wp-content/uploads/2012/09/KPStories-v1-no7-Sustainable-FINAL.pdf.
7. Jessica Trowbridge, "Food Matters: In Hospitals and for Prenatal Health," Environmental Health Policy Institute, http://www.psr.org/environment-and-health/environmental-health-policy-institute/responses/food-matters-in-hospitals-and-for-prenatal-health.html.
8. R. Sturm, "Childhood Obesity: What We Can Learn from Existing Data on Societal Trends, Part 2," *Preventing Chronic Disease* 2, no. 2 (2005), A20, http://www.ncbi.nlm.nih.gov/pubmed/15888231.
9. USDA Economic Research Service, "Nutrient Availability Documentation," http://www.ers.usda.gov/data-products/food-availability-%28per capita%29-data-system/nutrient-availability-documentation.aspx#.UuaoovbTnVo.
10. USDA Economic Research Service, "Data Sets: Food Expenditures," http://www.ers.usda.gov/data-products/food-expenditures.aspx#26636.
11. Stephanie Strom, "FDA Offers Broad New Rules to Fight Food Contamination," *New York Times*, January 5, 2013, A1.
12. Jamie Harvey, interviewed by the author.
13. "Is Processed Food a Pandora's Box for the American Diet? An Interview with Melanie Warner, author of *America Pandora's Lunchbox: How Processed Food Took over the American Meal*," *PBS News Hour*, April 29, 2013.

14. US Bureau of Labor Statistics. "American Time Use Survey: Household Activities, 2011," http://www.bls.gov/tus/current/household.htm (accessed November 15, 2013).

15. US CDC, "Basics About Childhood Obesity: How Is Childhood Overweight and Obesity Measured?" http://www.cdc.gov/obesity/childhood/basics.html.

16. Health Care Without Harm, "Chemicals in the Food System," http://www.healthy-foodinhealthcare.org/chemicals.foodsystem.php.

17. Patrice Sutton et al., "Reproductive Health and the Industrialized Food System: A Point of Intervention for Health Policy," *Health Affairs* 30, no. 5 (May 2011): 888–897.

18. Council on Environmental Health, American Academy of Pediatrics, "Pesticide Exposure in Children," *Pediatrics* 130, no. 6 (December 1, 2012): 1757–1763.

19. Quoted in Sutton. "Reproductive Health and the Industrialized Food System," 889.

20. Sturges D. Payne et al., "Evaluating Cumulative Organophosphorus Pesticide Body Burden of Children: A National Case Study," *Environmental Science & Technology* 43, no. 20 (2009): 7924–7930.

21. Sutton, "Reproductive Health and the Industrial Food System."

22. Ibid.

23. Patrick Heffer and Michel Prud'homme, "Short-Term Fertilizer Outlook, 2012–2013," November 2012, http://www.fertilizer.org/ifa/HomePage/LIBRARY/Publication-database.html/Short-Term-Fertilizer-Outlook-2012-2013.html.

24. Sutton, "Reproductive Health and the Industrialized Food System," 890.

25. Ibid.

26. US CDC, "Antibiotic Resistance Threats in the United States, 2013," http://www.cdc.gov/drugresistance/threat-report-2013/pdf/ar-threats-2013-508.pdf#page=6.

27. Thomas Newman, interviewed by the author.

28. Deborah Fleischer, "UCSF Academic Senate Approves Resolution to Phase Out Meat Raised with Non-Therapeutic Antibiotics," USF Living Green, May 2013, http://sustainability.ucsf.edu/1.353.

29. US Department of Health and Human Services, *Report on Carcinogens*, 12th edition (Washington, DC: HHS, 2011), http://ntp.niehs.nih.gov/ntp/roc/twelfth/profiles/Styrene.pdf.

30. Kaiser Permanente Division of Research, "In Utero Exposure to BPA May Adversely Affect Male Genital Development," press release, August 29, 2011, http://www.dor.kaiser.org/external/news/press_releases/In_Utero_exposure_to_BPA_May_Adversely_Affect_Male_Genital_Development/.

31. Zero Breast Cancer, "Phthalates (THAL-ates): The Everywhere Chemical," http://www.niehs.nih.gov/research/supported/assets/docs/j_q/phthalates_the_everywhere_chemical_handout_.pdf; Sarah Janssen, NRDC Switchboard, "What's for Lunch? Likely a Few Hormone-Disrupting Chemicals: Phthalates and BPA," http://switchboard.nrdc.org/blogs/sjanssen/whats_for_lunch_likely_a_few_h.html; Physicians for Social Responsibility, "Environmental Endocrine Disruptors: What Health Care Providers Should Know," http://www.psr.org/assets/pdfs/environmental-endocrine.pdf.

32. S. J. Vermeulen, B. M. Campbell, and J. S. I. Ingram, "Climate Change and Food Systems," *Annual Review of Environmental Resources* 37 (2012): 195–222; Natasha

Gilbert, "One-Third of Our Greenhouse Gas Emissions Come from Agriculture," *Nature*, October 31, 2012, http://www.nature.com/news/one-third-of-our-greenho use-gas-emissions-come-from-agriculture-1.11708.

33. P. Thornton, "Recalibrating Food Production in the Developing World: Global Warming Will Change More Than Just the Climate," CCAFS Policy Brief no. 6. (CGIAR Research Program on Climate Change, Agriculture and Food Security, 2012).

34. Kaiser Permanente Institute for Health Policy, "A Health Sector Guide to Food System and Agriculture Policy," *In Focus* 6 (fall 2009): 2–3.

35. Tom J. Thompson interviewed by Judith Nemes.

36. Addie Gibson interviewed by Nemes.

37. Lena Brook, Balanced Menus Evaluation 2010, presentation, San Francisco Bay Area Chapter, Physicians for Social Responsibility, http://www.psr.org/chapters/ oregon/healthy-food-in-health-care/balanced-menus-presentation.pdf.

38. Oregon Healthy Food in Health Care Newsletter, September/October 2010, http://www.psr.org/chapters/oregon/health-care-without-harm/healthy-food-in-health-care-newsletter/newsletters/hfhc-septemberoctober-2010.html.

39. St. Elizabeth's Medical Center, "St. E's, Boston Hospitals Showcase Success in Reducing Sugar-Sweetened Beverage Consumption," February 23, 2012, http://steward.org/ news/St-Elizabeths/St-Es-Boston-Hospitals-Showcase-Success-in-Reducing-Su gar-Sweetened-Beverage-Consumption.

40. Meghan Pierce, "Dartmouth-Hitchcock Medical Center Won't Sell Sugar-Sweetened Drinks," *New Hampshire Union Leader*, December 29, 2011, http://www.union-leader.com/article/20111230/NEWS07/712309991/0/opinion.

5

Managing and Minimizing Hospital Waste

When I began my job in environmental stewardship at Kaiser Permanente, one of the initial goals we set for our program was to minimize the volume and toxicity of waste. I decided that the best way to understand what we were up against was to get my hands dirty. Literally. I began a year-long tour of our 30 hospitals (now 38) and, with local staff, conducted "waste audits." That is a fancy way of saying we looked in trash cans and biohazardous waste containers. I counted containers and noted where they were placed, I spoke to hundreds of frontline workers and physicians about how they dispose of wastes, and—wearing safety gear—I followed waste from the point of generation to final disposal, including traveling to many of the local landfills. The best part of this experience was hearing creative ideas from staff about reducing wastes. Some told me they took recyclables home or to a school because they could not bear to throw them away. Others drew pictures of types of waste to be recycled and posted them on facility walls where the recycling containers should go. Many sought me out to say how much they wanted to see our performance improve. What I thought would be a dirty grind turned out to be a rewarding and enlightening experience.

HEALTH CARE'S WASTEFUL WAYS

Anyone who works in health care or wants to understand how it operates should spend some time at the back door of a hospital. There, in the hospital's underbelly, one can observe a constant stream of trash—from bottles, cans, and cardboard, to pharmaceuticals, sharps, and used lab solvents. At many hospitals, you will also hear the regular humming of the autoclave, a giant furnace-like apparatus that steam-sterilizes medical waste all day and night, preparing it to go to a landfill. But that is not all. Containers of hazardous waste, such as expired chemicals, chemotherapy, spent silver and lead, and diesel oil await pickup from specialized handlers. It is a surprising and even shocking scene to some, and one that goes on at every hospital across the country.

As health care providers, we are responsible for promoting health. Yet, in the process of delivering health care, US hospitals produce more than 2.3 million tons of waste annually.[1] That means hospitals generate an average of 26 pounds of waste per staffed bed in the course of a day. The US health care sector is second only to the food industry in contributing to waste production. Clearly, hospitals have a garbage problem.

Although other environmental issues garner more attention and publicity, no other initiative is more fundamental to building and sustaining environmentally responsible health care at the facility level than effective waste management. In fact, reduction of mercury-containing wastes and total hospital wastes were the top two of ten health care pollution mitigation goals set out in a landmark 1998 memorandum of understanding between the American Hospital Association and the US Environmental Protection Agency (EPA). Many hospitals have made impressive progress in this area, but even 15 years after the signing of the agreement, hospital waste of all kinds remains a major, costly problem, financially, environmentally, and in terms of human health. And, ironically, waste remains one of the lowest hanging, unpicked fruits in the greening of health care. "We speak to hospitals every day that are making a lot of progress in managing their waste," says Janet Howard, director of facility engagement at Practice Greenhealth. "But there are still others who haven't even started recycling yet."

Wastes Are a Plural Problem

In many ways, the movement to green the health care sector started with the problem of waste. Gary Cohen, who founded Health Care Without Harm with colleague Charlotte Brody in 1996, remembers reading a US EPA report citing hospital incinerators as the country's number-one source of carcinogenic dioxin emissions. He asked himself: How could the industry that existed to heal people be doing so much harm? In answering that question over the following decade, Cohen and Brody and Health Care Without Harm made great progress in reducing, but not eliminating, the health and environmental costs of medical waste incineration. And they also found out that the incineration of wastes was just the tip of the iceberg of a much greater, more varied issue involving many very different types of wastes, each of which was associated with unique health or environmental problems, and each of which demanded its own solutions.

"What makes this issue so challenging is the sheer volume of different waste materials we deal with every day," says Michael Geller, regional sustainability manager for Providence Health and Services in Portland, Oregon. "We also face the perception that the waste is dirty and infectious." But while hospitals have perhaps the most complex waste streams of any industry—plastics, chemicals, paper, food, needles, drugs, chemicals, medical devices, radioactive materials, packaging, and, increasingly, large quantities of electronics, the vast majority is not toxic. As much as 80 to 85 percent of the overall waste is comparable to domestic waste (see Fig. 5.1). The remaining 15 to 20 percent, however, is considered hazardous and may be infectious, toxic, or radioactive. By focusing on waste that is not hazardous and that typically is sent to landfills, hospitals could reduce their operating costs by almost 20 percent by implementing the 4Rs:

- Reduce: Using environmentally preferable purchasing policies, purchase only the material and products that are needed.
- Reuse: Donate medical devices or use technologies like reprocessing to get multiple lives out of products and equipment.

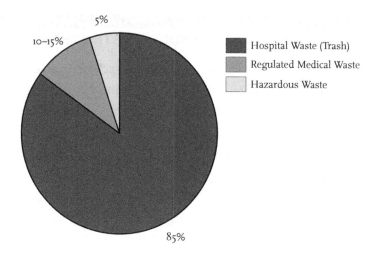

5%
10–15%

■ Hospital Waste (Trash)
■ Regulated Medical Waste
□ Hazardous Waste

85%

Figure 5.1
Main categories of hospital waste.
(SOURCE: Sustainability Roadmaps for Hospitals, www.sustainabilityroadmap.org/topics/
waste.shtml)

- Recycle: Divert all recyclable materials, such as paper, cardboard, glass, plastics and aluminum from the landfill.
- Rot: Compost materials such as food, green waste, and compostable service ware.

Segregation of Waste Streams

There is an important step before recycling: segregating waste streams to ensure that nonregulated waste like paper, cardboard glove boxes, drapes, and the like are recycled or disposed of as regular trash (see Box 5.1). Inova Health System, a nonprofit health care system based in Northern Virginia and Washington, DC, that serves more than 2 million people reduced its regulated medical waste (RMW) stream by more than 500 tons over 14 months, saving more than $250,000.[2] New York-Presbyterian Healthcare system was able to divert 900 tons of recyclables after developing a comprehensive waste management system in 2008.[3] By reducing its trash volume, it saw a savings of $10,000 per year.

Box 5.1 GETTING TO KNOW YOUR WASTE STREAMS

To set effective waste management goals and track performance, it is important to uncover details on the types, amounts, and associated costs for material disposal.[4] That requires, at a minimum, recognizing one type of waste from another.

- **Solid waste:** Also called municipal waste, black bag, clear bag, or nonregulated waste. This is general trash, similar to what you would find in a hotel but with more plastics and packaging. The typical cost range for disposing this waste is .03–$ 0.08 per pound (costs vary by geographic location).
- **Regulated medical waste (RMW):** Also called potentially infectious material, red bag waste or biohazardous waste. RMW is regulated state by state but also falls under OSHA's Blood borne Pathogen Standard. The typical cost range for this waste is .20–.50 per pound.
- **RCRA hazardous waste:** Hazardous waste is defined and regulated by the US EPA under the Resource Conservation and Recovery Act (RCRA) and is either a "listed" waste or meets the characteristics of a hazardous waste. Additionally, some states have promulgated regulations that further define and regulate hazardous waste. Common RCRA hazardous wastes include hazardous pharmaceuticals, bulk chemotherapeutic agents, mercury, xylene, and other solvents, some paints, aerosol cans, and other products. The typical disposal cost range for this waste is $1.70–$2.00 per pound.
- **Pharmaceutical waste:** Some pharmaceutical waste is RCRA hazardous, though most may not require handling as hazardous waste; however, it should receive special disposal considerations to prevent contaminating groundwater. Additionally, controlled substances such as narcotics must be disposed of in accordance with federal Drug Enforcement Agency requirements. Disposal costs vary depending on the disposal mechanism.

- **Universal waste:** This is a confusing category but one worth learning about. Under the US EPA's rules, generators of some hazardous wastes, including batteries, mercury-containing devices like thermostats, light bulbs, and certain pesticides, *may be* managed under a less stringent set of regulations in order to facilitate more streamlined recycling efforts. States can set their own requirements, and many do. The typical cost range for this waste is $ 0.75–$1.00 per pound.
- **Recyclables:** Recyclables are items and materials that can be converted into a reusable material. Recyclables in health care include the usual suspects found in commercial buildings such as paper, cardboard, beverage and food containers, metal, and glass. The typical cost range for this waste stream is.01 per pound.
- **Construction and demolition debris (C&D):** This waste stream comprises bulky material like ceiling tiles, plumbing fixtures, carpeting, concrete, bricks, and fill dirt generated during construction and renovation projects. Recycling of C&D waste is a common consideration in new construction and renovation projects, as it can qualify the organization for points under LEED certification or the *Green Guide for Healthcare.*
- **Composting:** This waste stream primarily comprises food and landscaping waste—material that will break down naturally and quickly, such as grass, weed clippings, tree limbs and branches, waste from vegetable produce, bread and grains, and paper products such as napkins or paper plates. One hospital found that 23 percent of its total waste stream was food waste. Organizations are finding ways to compost this material—either onsite or using an offsite contractor. Diverting this waste from solid waste can significantly reduce waste disposal costs.

Segregation of nonregulated waste from the RMW stream can be challenging. The Healthcare Environmental Resource Center suggests the following measures, some of which are mandated by state or federal environmental or health and safety regulations:

- Use separate, color-coded and labeled RMW collection containers (e.g., red bags and sharps containers).
- Post signs in multiple languages as necessary, at RMW disposal locations outlining what types of waste are to be disposed of as RMW.
- Determine waste generation rates for specific areas of the hospital and provide appropriately sized containers for those areas.
- Where RMW containers are used, also provide regular waste containers to ensure that employees are making a conscious disposal and segregation decision.
- Cover red bag containers to reduce solid waste that is casually tossed in.
- Do not provide red bags in areas where RMW is not generated.
- Train all employees on RMW segregation. Reinforce waste segregation as part of annual training requirements.
- Track RMW generation by department and hold department heads accountable for their RMW generation and disposal costs.
- Track progress, report success, and reward staff for their efforts.

THE HEALTH AND ENVIRONMENTAL CONSEQUENCES OF WASTE

Concern about hospital waste is not simply a bottom-line issue (although it is clearly a major cost in health care). Even more important, waste can be toxic to human and environmental health, and health care organizations have a compelling responsibility to limit it to the least amount possible.

Broadly speaking, the health and environmental consequences of disposing of the many types of waste include the following:

- Cancer and developmental and reproductive effects caused by the release of toxins—notably dioxins and mercury—from medical and solid waste incinerators.[5]
- Human health hazards and explosions caused by the generation of methane gas from the decomposition of organic materials in landfills.[6]
- Global warming and other climate change caused in part by the emission of greenhouse gases from traditional methods of waste disposal.[7]

Although it is true that most hospital waste is nonhazardous, non-infectious solid waste or trash (paper, cardboard, plastics), most of it—what is not recycled—ultimately ends up in a landfill, where it produces methane. Landfills are the third largest source of methane emissions in the United States, and pound for pound, the impact of methane on climate change is more than 20 times greater than carbon dioxide over a 100-year period.[8] Methane seeps from decomposing organic materials in landfills into the air, and it can even seep through underground pathways into nearby buildings. Over the years, a number of landfills have been the sites of spontaneous methane explosions, some harming nearby residents.[9] The US EPA's Office of Solid Waste and Emergency Response found that 42 percent of all US greenhouse gases emitted in 2006 were associated with the manufacturing, use, and disposal of materials and products, the majority of which were nonhazardous and noninfectious.[10]

Biohazardous and hazardous wastes that end up in incinerators also produce greenhouse gas emissions, as well as releases of dioxins, heavy metals such as mercury and cadmium, hydrogen chloride gas, and other toxic substances, including PCBs and furans. Incinerators actually emit more carbon dioxide per megawatt-hour than any fossil fuel–based power source, including coal-fired power plants.[11]

It is good news that rates of incineration of hospital wastes have decreased dramatically across the country over the past decade, but we still have a way to go. Stericycle, the largest medical waste handler in the United States, still operates several large incinerators, in part because some wastes are required by law to be treated with very high heat.

The release of toxic substances in incineration is especially prevalent when wastes are burned at low temperatures, or when plastics that contain polyvinyl chloride (PVC) are included in the mix. Dioxins, furans, and heavy metals all persist for long periods in the environment, and they are bioaccumulative over time. Most of us have it in our bodies.[12] In humans, dioxins have the potential to cause cancer and to produce a broad spectrum of adverse effects because they can alter the fundamental growth and development of cells, weaken the immune system, and interfere with the endocrine system, which is responsible for making hormones needed to regulate bodily functions, including sexual development and fertility.[13]

HOW HEALTH CARE IS RESPONDING

Getting Started: Creating a Waste Management Plan

Probably the most effective way to reduce the environmental and health impacts of hospital waste disposal is to focus not on the end of the process but the beginning by reducing the amount of waste the health care facility generates in the first place. It is not an easy task, but one—or rather many tasks—that hundreds of hospitals are focusing on across the country and even the world.

Health Care Without Harm put it well: "The less regulated medical waste (RMW) there is, the more solid waste. The less solid waste, the more recyclables. The less products that are purchased, the less total waste to dispose of." For example, it has been estimated that reducing 1 ton of office paper by source reduction (rather than recycling or incineration) will eliminate an estimated 8 tons of greenhouse gas equivalents (counting both the reduced emissions from less paper plus the pollutants avoided from the paper's manufacture, transport, and disposal).[14] Source reduction sounds straightforward, but it is no silver bullet. Rather, a broad range of activities and approaches can collectively make a dent, including smarter purchasing, better segregation of waste to improve recycling rates, a focus on the operating room, reprocessing of single-use medical devices, and even more comprehensive recycling of electronics and construction debris.

But first, do some planning. It may be tempting for a newly created green team to launch into any one or more of the aforementioned activities, but carefully and methodically planning your program at the outset will go far in ensuring that you accomplish your goals. The Sustainability Roadmap for Hospitals project, a joint endeavor of the American Society for Healthcare Engineering (ASHE), the Association for the Healthcare Environment (AHE), and the Association for Healthcare Resource & Materials Management (AHRMM) of the American Hospital Association, suggests the following 10 steps for creating a comprehensive waste management plan:

- **Understand your waste streams:** For each waste stream—solid waste, RMW, hazardous waste, and the like—understand all federal and state regulatory considerations, as well as who is internally responsible for each stream, how each is handled, what are the policies and procedures, and who are the waste haulers.
- **Measure/baseline current waste generation**: Establishing waste stream baselines is an important first step in tracking progress. You cannot measure what you do not know you have, nor can you set reasonable goals or report on successes.
- **Complete a facility-wide waste operations assessment**: Internally, assess waste and recycling container placement, color coding, labeling, and utilization to maximize efficiencies and reduce costs and transportation impacts.
- **Build multi-stakeholder teams and get leadership support:** Creating a green team with representatives from all departments that share responsibility for the purchase, management, and/or

disposal of particular waste streams is key. If possible, dedicate resources toward a waste minimization coordinator.

- **Set targets/goals:** Set both short- and long-term reduction goals for waste minimization and integrate them into a meaningful and achievable waste management plan. The Healthier Hospitals Initiative's three-level challenge for waste reduction is a great place to start (see Box 5.2). Target setting allows an organization to establish reasonable goals that are consistent with a basic, intermediate or advanced approach.

- **Develop strategic action plans for improvement:** Pick and choose specific projects, such as reducing RMW waste generation or switching to reusable sharps containers, which help you meet your overall goals.

- **Ensure regulatory compliance across all waste streams:** This is not optional.

- **Adopt and record integrated waste management policies and procedures** for each and every waste stream.

- **Track, measure, and report:** It is important to begin to track waste reduction measures for several reasons: (1) to verify they are meeting the intended goal, (2) to track cost and operational savings, (3) to monitor staff satisfaction, and (4) to report on all of these successes, or failures, to inform your next steps.

- **Train, educate, and celebrate:** Involved staff must be educated both formally and informally of the reasons for any changes, trained on work practice changes, and informed with ongoing feedback on how the action plan's progress is meeting the goals. Never let a success go unrecognized.[15]

Taking Action: Major Hospital Waste Streams

Once a waste-focused green team has done its planning, including a comprehensive waste assessment, it should be a relatively easy matter to prioritize

---

> Box 5.2 **THE HEALTHIER HOSPITALS INITIATIVE'S WASTE CHALLENGE**
>
> The Healthier Hospitals Initiative's progressive, three-level challenge to participating hospitals on waste reduction includes the following:
> - **RMW reduction**: Reduce RMW to either less than 10 percent of total waste or less than 3 pounds per adjusted patient day.
> - **Recycling**: Recycle 15 percent of total waste.
> - **C&D diversion**: Implement a construction and demolition debris recycling program for major renovations and new construction to achieve at least 80 percent recycle and diversion rate.

---

a list of targets, since the team will have identified all the areas of low-cost, high-payoff opportunities. For many hospitals, especially those with in-house expertise in smarter, greener product purchasing, there is no better place to operationalize a waste reduction plan than the operating room.

TARGETING THE OPERATING ROOM

Despite the small footprint of operating rooms (ORs) in the typical hospital, they account for as much as 42 percent of all patient-related income and 33 percent of all supply costs.[16] They are also major energy hogs, as well as being hospitals' number-one source of high-cost regulated medical waste and as much as 30 percent of all hospital waste, more than half of which is composed of single-use disposable items.[17]

In 2011, a team from Johns Hopkins University Hospital conducted a review of the medical literature over an 8-year period to identify the greatest opportunities for waste reduction in surgical suites. They noted that hospital operating rooms were notorious for disposing of unused but open sterilized equipment, using energy-sucking overhead lights, and failing to segregate harmless waste from hazardous waste.

The team, led by Martin A. Makary, MD, an associate professor of surgery at the John Hopkins University School of Medicine, worked with a panel of experts on hospital environmental practices to identify the most practical strategies for reducing OR waste. Their top five recommendations were as follows:

- Reduce and segregate OR waste.
- Reprocess single-use medical devices (SUDs).
- Make environmentally preferable purchasing decisions.
- Manage OR energy consumption.
- Manage pharmacy waste.

They noted that as much as 90 percent of what ends up in red bags (for regulated medical waste) does not meet the criteria for regulated waste and could be far more cheaply disposed of as regular trash.[18]

In 2010, Practice Greenhealth launched its Greening the OR Initiative to help hospitals focus on OR waste as one of the most achievable ways of reducing costs and environmental impacts, while improving or maintaining worker and patient health and safety. More than 300 hospitals and health systems have since endorsed the initiative and are adopting a series of OR best practices, beginning with HHI's focus on reducing the extraneous contents of OR surgical kits and purchasing reprocessed single-use devices for reuse. A third approach, purchasing reusable or recyclable rather than disposable products, is also increasingly common.

Reformulating Operating Room Packs

Many of the medical devices and other products used in surgical procedures arrive in the OR as sterilized, prepackaged kits formulated specifically for dozens of kinds of surgical procedures. They contain everything from surgical tools like drill bits, saws, blades, biopsy forceps, syringes, and endoscopic scissors to plastic basins and cups, Styrofoam trays, gauze dressing, plastic tubing, and towels. And every kit comes wrapped in blue wrap, a hard-to-recycle packaging material made of #5 polypropylene plastic.

These kits often contain items that are rarely used during an operation, but once the sterile kit is opened, the unused items can no longer be considered sterile, per US FDA regulations, and must be disposed of.

Not infrequently, entire kits are opened and laid out for a procedure that ends up being cancelled. In many ORs, all the contents are tossed into the RMW bins, which costs five to ten times more than solid waste to dispose of and is linked to a variety of environmental hazards through treatment and disposal.[19] Many ORs mistakenly dispose of more than 50 percent of their waste, including the blue wrap and cardboard packaging, as RMW.[20]

To prevent this extravagance, OR green teams, including surgeons, infectious disease specialists, OR nurses, and representatives from purchasing and environmental services, can be trained to assess the various surgical kits for unnecessary items and advise procurement personnel to requisition packs that have been customized and standardized to meet their actual needs. This, of course, requires the participation and support of OR leadership and surgical staff, since there is typically a large variation in the kit contents preferred among different surgeons performing the same operation.

This is what the University of Minnesota Medical Center (UMMC), Fairview, did beginning in 2009 after Dr. Rafael Andrade, a general thoracic surgeon, got curious about the amount of OR waste from surgical kits. Andrade, who made the case for reformulating surgical kits at Practice Greenhealth's inaugural workshop on Greening the OR in 2010, closely examined how he and other surgeons used a kit for port placement procedures for chemotherapy patients, a procedure performed several hundred times a year at UMMC. He found he could reduce the number of items in the kit from 44 to 27 without impacting surgeon preferences. By reformulating the contents of that single kit he found he could reduce the amount of items going off to landfills or incineration by about 80 pounds a year, saving UMMC around $2,000 in unnecessary product purchases and disposal costs.

Andrade took his kit reformulation experiment to the next level by enlisting the hospital's first green team to look for seldom-used items in 38 additional OR kits, gather input from the surgical staff on content revisions, and negotiate with the OR kit vendors to remove those items and lower the kit prices. Reformulating a kit for thoracotomy surgery ended up reducing more than 600 pounds of waste and saving more than $12,000 a year. In all, UMMC's kit reformulations at two campuses produced more than 10,000 pounds of waste reduction and saved the system more than $116,000 annually, not counting the savings from avoided RMW or solid waste disposal.[21]

Mayo Clinic implemented a similar review process at about the same time, enlisting OR staff, the procurement team, and surgical kit suppliers to find ways to reduce the inventory overage while still meeting the needs and preferences of surgeons. According to Kevin Hoyde, a consultant in Mayo's supply chain management system, the savings amounted to more than $125,000 within the first few years while greatly reducing the amount of material being carted off to landfills or incinerators.[22]

RECYCLING BLUE WRAP

Kaiser Permanente zeroed in on another aspect of the problem by focusing on the 679,000 pounds of blue wrap we purchase each year at a cost of about $2 million to maintain the sterility of medical instruments. The problem with blue wrap disposal is that it has a relatively low recycling value and is otherwise costly and cumbersome to manage.

Over a 3-year period, our sourcing director and other operations leaders pressed our blue wrap supplier to find a recycling solution for their product. They eventually agreed to accept responsibility for finding recyclers for 75 percent of our blue wrap purchase by 2011, diverting 510,000 pounds of plastic and almost 45,000 pounds of cardboard from landfills and avoiding $94,000 in disposal costs.[23] Going forward, some facilities are switching from blue wrap to reusable aluminum containers.

REPROCESSING SINGLE-USE DEVICES

Another way to reduce OR waste, save money, and limit environmental pollution is to recycle so-called disposable SUDs. At third-party reprocessors, they are cleaned, function-tested, repackaged, sterilized and then resold to the hospital at a steeply discounted price. More than 100 devices labeled as SUDs can be reprocessed and reused, including such common items as trocars, ultrasonic scalpels, compression devices, diagnostic ultrasound catheters, drill bits, saws, forceps, and laparoscopic and endo-scopic scissors.

Not so long ago, many of these and other medical devices were made of durable materials, like stainless steel, glass, or rubber, and could be repro-cessed after use by the hospital's own sterile processing department and thus reused multiple times. That began to change back in the 1980s due to concerns in the early days of AIDS about infection control and sterility, especially in the OR environment. Medical device manufacturers took ad-vantage of the concerns by producing plastic, disposable devices and label-ing almost everything as "single use," even for products that were similar or identical to the previously reusable devices. Today, the market for dis-posable medical supplies in the United States is booming at $37.8 billion a year (as of 2012), growing by 4.3 percent annually—a major driver in the growth of the greater than 6-million-ton mountain of waste generated by US hospitals every year.[24]

However, since the late 1990s, a new service industry has come along to make a significant dent in the disposables market by collecting and reprocessing many of these devices labeled for single use (an industry label not required by the FDA). Although the original equipment mak-ers have fought back by warning surgeons that reprocessed SUDs may be unsafe or of inferior quality, the FDA has taken steps since 2000 to re-quire that reprocessing companies meet the same quality and safety stan-dards as those applied to original equipment manufacturers. The FDA has found no evidence that reprocessing has caused any health risks—a con-clusion reaffirmed by a 2008 report to Congress by the US Government Accountability Office (GAO).[25] From 1997 to 2007, the new industry safely reprocessed more than 50 million devices and prevented more than 10,000 tons of medical waste from entering landfills.[26]

Today, the purchase of reprocessed SUDs is common practice among the nation's top hospitals. An FDA survey in 2009 found that 25 percent of more than 6,000 hospitals and outpatient surgery centers use at least one kind of reprocessed SUD.

For instance, in a 12-month period in 2010–2011, Johns Hopkins University Hospital saved nearly $1.2 million by reprocessing SUDs.[27]

Michigan's Metro Health Hospital, which serves the Grand Rapids area, began reprocessing SUDs from its 10 ORs in 2008 and over the next 3 years realized a savings of more than $235,000 in purchasing costs while avoiding nearly 2 tons of waste.[28] Advocate Christ Medical Center in Oak Lawn, Illinois, saved $400,000 and avoided sending nearly 5 tons of waste to the incinerator or landfills in 2010 alone.[29] In fact, the vast majority of Practice Greenhealth's 149 award winners in 2012 collectively diverted more than 333 tons of medical waste by SUD reprocessing at a total savings of more than $18 million.[30]

Kaiser Permanente accounted for a large portion of that total. In 2011, we increased annual SUD reprocessing to 173 tons of potential waste, up from 27 tons in 2003, and avoided an estimated $8.2 million in purchasing and waste disposal costs.[31] In addition, we avoided costs by switching from disposable to reusable products for surgical basins and surgical textiles such as gowns and table drapes.

One does not usually think of surgical gowns and table drapes as "devices," but the FDA does, and it enforces strict safety and quality standards on their use for protection against the transfer of microorganisms or body fluids. Because those standards could not have been met by the surgical textiles in use 30 years ago, nearly all hospitals switched to new disposable products with lower upfront costs.[32]

Today, however, reusable surgical textiles meet or exceed the barrier protection standards of the Association for the Advancement of Medical Instrumentation, and many leading hospitals have switched back to reusables, which can reduce OR waste by up to 80 percent and cost less than disposables over their lifetime.[33] A 2009 life-cycle analysis study of reusable textiles at the University of Minnesota Medical Center, Fairview, in collaboration with the Minnesota Technical Assistance Program, concluded that switching from disposable to reusable gowns avoided 254,000 pounds of waste and saved $360,000 a year, with no difference in infection prevention attributes.[34] Additionally, over their lifetimes, the reusables resulted in three times less carbon dioxide emissions than disposables and sixteen times less carcinogenic emissions.

Kaiser Permanente compared the clinical performance, total cost, and environmental impacts of reusables versus disposables and found that by switching out just 100,000 from the 800,000 surgical gowns used annually from disposable to reusable could eliminate nearly 22.5 tons of waste and save nearly $10,000 in disposal costs while also simplifying the supply chain management operations. On the basis of that finding, it awarded a national contract for reusable gowns.

REUSABLE SHARPS CONTAINERS

Every year, health care facilities throw away thousands of tons of plastic in the form of disposable sharps containers. Hospitals then pay a premium to treat the containers as regulated medical waste. Disposal of regulated medical waste means some of the plastic components are incinerated, releasing a host of toxic substances having negative impacts on human health and the environment.

Disposal of sharps containers has been associated with as much as 13 percent of the total sharps injuries inside a hospital. One study found replacing disposable sharps containers with reusable ones reduced sharps injuries by 33 percent by eliminating overfilling of the containers.[35]

Being reusable as many as 500 times, reusable sharps containers have several environmental benefits, including the following:

- Reducing the manufacture of new containers and associated greenhouse gas; emissions from reduced manufacturing, packaging, and transportation.
- Reducing medical waste by 3.5 tons for every 100 beds and cardboard waste by 1 ton for every 300 beds.

The Harvard Medical School has two large research buildings constituting its North Campus that fully transitioned from the use of disposable to reusable plastic sharps containers in 2009. In the first year of the program, the project reduced 6,774 pounds of plastic from the waste stream and was cost neutral.[36]

Box 5.3 WHEN WASTE IS WANTED

One country's health care trash is often another's treasure. Over the past two decades, several nonprofit organizations have sprung up to fill an important need. These organizations, such as Georgia-based MedShare and Ohio-based MedWish, collect excess medical supplies and equipment and send them to the developing world and locations in need of emergency medical materials. They also outfit medical missions and safety net clinics in both the United States and abroad.

The organizations perform an important social mission, but they also help prevent a significant amount of waste. To date, MedWish has recovered more than 2.2 million pounds of medical surplus from over 50 hospitals in the United States. In 2011, MedWish diverted more than 500,000 pounds of usable medical surplus from disposal, keeping these life-saving items out of landfills and putting them in the hands of people in need. MedShare, for its part, has obtained and shared more than $93 million worth of life-saving medical supplies and equipment since the organization was founded in 1999.

Recycling and Reusing Electronic Devices

As anyone who has recently been inside a hospital or doctor's office can attest, the medical profession is in the midst of a digital revolution. As hospitals across the country gear up for the digital requirements of the Affordable Care Act, they are also facing—along with every other industry—the dilemma of what to do about a growing tide of electronics waste that accompanies an increased reliance on computers and other electronics (see Box 5.3). Some large-scale recycling practices—primarily in China, India, Nigeria, and Vietnam—expose recycling workers and surrounding communities to toxic chemicals in the discarded products. Among the most troubling e-waste pollutants are lead, mercury, cadmium, barium, beryllium, phosphorus, and brominated flame retardants.[37]

However, these are not the entire story. Today's electronics—including many medical devices—contain four minerals that, when sourced from the Democratic Republic of Congo (DRC), may be associated with serious human rights abuses there.[38] Documenting the source of gold, tungsten, tantalum, and tin is now required of suppliers by legislation enacted in August 2012.[39]

Thanks to a partnership with Redemtech (now called Arrow Value Recovery), a technology recycler that that is a certified e-Stewards® recycler, Kaiser Permanente has committed to exporting zero waste by recycling all of our discarded electronic devices while ensuring that all Protected Health Information on devices is purged from any digital asset before it is resold or recycled. Through this partnership, hundreds of thousands of pounds of retired Kaiser Permanente technology devices—desktop and laptop computers, servers, handheld devices of all sorts—have been resold to be used by another organization or rendered into raw materials and sold nationwide to various industries as raw material.

In 2013, for instance, Kaiser Permanente recycled or reused more than 187,000 pieces of electronic equipment weighing about 1,016 tons.

For equipment that cannot be repaired, refurbished, or upgraded, Redemtech harvests serviceable parts to repair other equipment. When nothing usable is left, it uses e-Stewards certified downstream recycling processors to return every recoverable commodity to the manufacturing stream. Mercury handlers reclaim the mercury, leaded glass heads to the lead smelter, and plastic to the plastic recycler. No electronic waste is ever sent to a landfill, nothing is ever incinerated, and no nonfunctioning equipment is ever shipped abroad. In total, the company has ethically processed more than 1.4 million devices for Kaiser Permanente.

RECYCLING CONSTRUCTION DEBRIS

Amid the daunting challenges of the health care waste stream, another bright spot has emerged: recycling of construction debris. This is especially important in California, where 29 percent of the volume of landfill waste comes from construction and demolition debris.[40] The state's hospitals are contributing a good deal to that as they comply with seismic regulations that have led to the replacement of 800 hospital buildings across the state.

Kaiser Permanente is one of those California-based hospital systems in the midst of seismic retrofits and full hospital construction projects. With recycling in mind, we have been working with our contractors to meet local municipalities' waste diversion requirements, which in most cities is 50 percent of construction debris. However, in many cases we exceed these standards, and it is not unusual for us to recycle nearly 100 percent of construction debris at our major projects. During construction of a 264-bed, six-story hospital in San Leandro, for instance, we recycled virtually all building materials, diverting 85,000 tons of waste from landfills and saving an estimated $817,000. While building our new Los Angeles medical center, we recycled 97 percent of construction debris during a major renovation. And during the equipment phase of building a new hospital in Modesto—when an enormous amount of shrink wrap, bubble wrap, cardboard, wooden pallets, and other packaging materials from manufacturers showed up—we managed to send just one dumpster of trash to the landfill while diverting 40 tons of waste.

CASE STUDIES: HEALTHY SOLUTIONS TO WASTE

Greening the Operating Room at Metro West Medical Center

Metro West Medical Center in Framingham, Massachusetts, was one of just four health systems inducted into Practice Greenhealth's prestigious Environmental Leadership Circle in 2012.[41] A teaching hospital and the largest health care provider in the region between Boston and Worcester, Metro West's sustainability committee, under the leadership of Dr. Amy Collins, decided in 2010 to take on the problem of the excessive cost and environmental impacts of blue sterilization wrap, which they estimated made up nearly 20 percent of the waste in Metro West's 16 surgical rooms. What makes blue wrap a particularly costly waste is the fact that it frequently is incorrectly disposed of in bins for regulated medical waste instead of those for solid waste, which is far cheaper to dispose of. Metro

West's solution was to phase out most blue wrap for instrument sterilization and instead to purchase several hundred rigid, reusable hard cases
for two thirds of its surgical procedures. The switch to reusable containers saved the hospital nearly $30,000 in avoided blue wrap purchases and
disposal fees in the first year and reduced its waste stream by more than
5,600 pounds of blue wrap alone. The 10-year projected savings is more
than $230,000.

Providence St. Vincent Medical Center

St. Vincent Medical Center in Portland, Oregon, a part of the big five-state
Providence Health and Services system, has made its annual staff barbeque
into a fitting, if unusual, symbol of its commitment to the elimination of
waste. Beginning in 2006, sustainability leader Michael Geller, who had already launched an ambitious recycling program at the hospital, decided to
boost staff awareness about waste by holding a "zero waste" barbecue. The
first year, he says, about 600 people came out for the barbecue, where they
enjoyed an outdoor feast of the usual hot dogs, hamburgers, beverages, chips,
and other goodies. What was unusual was that virtually all of the food served
was locally produced, reducing transportation-related greenhouse gas emissions, and at the end of the day there was virtually no waste. Everything was
served in biodegradable, compostable containers, all food scraps went into
compost bins, and all edible food was donated to St. Vincent de Paul. By the
third year of the event, 3,500 staff showed up, with guests, and left behind
one single garbage can of true garbage—mostly candy bar wrappers.

St. Vincent's has taken conservation to new heights, winning multiple
awards from Practice Greenhealth for its efforts. It has reduced OR waste
by reprocessing single-use devices and ordering individually wrapped
medical instruments to avoid the waste associated with multipacks; it is
buying more and more products from local producers; and it is even striving to employ more local adults with disabilities to sort the materials from
the recycle bins in its own, in-house recycling center. The hospital sends
more than 3 tons of food waste per week to a local compost facility, but

only after they grind and dewater it in a machine to reduce its volume and weight. Their reusable sharps container program, adopted for environmental and safety reasons, has had the nice co-benefit of saving the hospital some $70,000 a year.

Looking ahead, Geller is working with a broader group of hospital representatives and the city of Portland to make a recycling service like this available to all Oregon hospitals.[42]

Kaiser Permanente: Setting a High Bar on Waste

Kaiser Permanente sets ambitious targets on green initiatives in every area of our sustainability agenda. Our system wide rate of waste reduction via reuse, recycling, and composting was 41 percent at the end of 2013, exceeding our 2015 target. This does not include construction and demolition debris, which is already recycled or reclaimed at rates above 90 percent.

To increase our rates further, Kaiser Permanente is looking broadly at our operations, especially seeking out innovative pilot programs that could be implemented system wide. A few of the best practices that are taking place include the following:

- In Los Angeles and Riverside, Kaiser Permanente medical centers have teamed up with unions to put hundreds of housekeeping and janitorial workers through "green jobs" training that allows them to do their jobs in more environmentally responsible ways.
- Participation in medical device recycling programs for items such as compression sleeves and ultrasonic scalpels avoided more than $9 million of costs in 2013 by reducing spending on both waste disposal and device purchasing.
- Many Kaiser Permanente hospitals throughout California have developed innovative programs to recycle or reuse blue wrap.
- Kaiser Permanente's partners are also helping to cut waste. MedShare, a key partner in medical supply recycling, was awarded the 2011 California Reuse Award for its work in providing recycled

medical supplies and equipment to safety-net clinics throughout California. Kaiser Permanente donated over 63,000 pounds of medical supplies and equipment to MedShare in 2010.

- Waste reduction goes far beyond recycling. Kaiser Permanente HealthConnect, the organization-wide electronic health record system, also helps preserve resources and trim waste. The organization achieved an annual recurring avoidance of at least 1,000 tons of paper waste and 100 tons of X-ray film waste by taking advantage of electronic health records to replace paper medical charts and by using digital X-ray technology.

NOTES

1. Gifty Kwakye, Gabriel A. Brat, and Martin A. Makary, "Green Surgical Practices for Health Care," *JAMA Archives of Surgery* 146, no. 2 (2011): 131–136.
2. Practice Greenhealth, "Inova Fairfax Hospital: Regulated Medical Waste Reduction and Minimization," Greening the OR Case Study, https://practicegreenhealth.org/ sites/default/files/upload-files/casestudy_inova_r6_web.pdf.
3. Bill Turpin and Linda D. Lee, "Waste Not: Developing a Hospital Recycling Program," *Health Facilities Management* (March 2012), http://www.hfmmagazine. com/hfmmagazine/jsp/articledisplay.jsp?dcrpath=HFMMAGAZINE/Article/ data/01JAN2011/0111HFM_FEA_enviro&domain=HFMMAGAZINE.
4. This section is adapted from Practice Greenhealth, "Waste Categories and Types," http://practicegreenhealth.org/topics/waste/waste-categories-types.
5. US EPA, "Persistent Bioaccumulative and Toxic (BPT) Chemical Program: Dioxins and Furans," http://www.epa.gov/pbt/pubs/dioxins.htm; US EPA, "Mercury: Health Effects," http://www.epa.gov/mercury/effects.htm.
6. Agency for Toxic Substances and Disease Registry, "Landfill Gas Primer, An Overview for Environmental Health Professionals: Chapter 3, Landfill Gas Safety and Health Issues," http://www.atsdr.cdc.gov/HAC/landfill/html/ch3.html.
7. US EPA, "Climate Change and Waste," http://epa.gov/climatechange/ climate-change-waste/.
8. US EPA, "Overview of Greenhouse Gases," http://epa.gov/climatechange/ghgemis-sions/gases/ch4.html.
9. Agency for Toxic Substances and Disease Registry, "Landfill Gas Primer: An Overview for Environmental Health Professionals," http://www.atsdr.cdc.gov/ HAC/landfill/html/intro.html.
10. US EPA, "Solid Waste Management and Greenhouse Gases," http://epa.gov/epa-waste/conserve/tools/warm/SWMGHGreport.html.
11. Global Alliance for Incinerator Alternatives, http://www.no-burn.org/section. php?id=84.

12. CDC, "Factsheet: Dioxins, Furans and Dioxin-Like Polychlorinated Biphenyls," http://www.cdc.gov/biomonitoring/DioxinLikeChemicals_FactSheet.html.

13. World Health Organization, "Dioxins and Their Effects on Human Health," http://www.who.int/mediacentre/factsheets/fs225/en/.

14. Catherine Zimmer, "Reducing the Detrimental Effects of Hospital Waste," *Health Facilities Management* (March 2012), http://www.hfmmagazine.com/hfmmagazine/jsp/articledisplay.jsp?dcrpath=HFMMAGAZINE/Article/data/03MAR2012/0312HFM_FEA_EnvironmentalServices&domain=HFMMAGAZINE.

15. This section is adapted from Sustainability Roadmap for Hospitals, http://www.sustainabilityroadmap.org/strategies/planwaste.shtml#.UpOWZyfOSkM.

16. McKesson Information Systems Inc. and the Healthcare Financial Management Association, "Achieving Operating Room Efficiency Through Process Integration," http://www.optimiumhealth.com/wp-resources/achieving-operating-room-efficiency-through-process-integration.pdf.

17. M. E. Tieszen and J. C. Gruenberg "A Quantitative, Qualitative and Critical Assessment of Surgical Waste, *JAMA* 267 (1992): 2765–2768.

18. Kwakye, Brat, and Makary, "Green Surgical Practices for Health Care."

19. Roy K. Esaki and Alex Macario "Wastage of Supplies and Drugs in the Operating Room," October 21, 2009, http://www.medscape.com/viewarticle/710513.

20. Practice Greenhealth and Greening the OR, "Implementation Module: Regulated Medical Waste Segregation and Minimization in the OR," https://practicegreenhealth.org/sites/default/files/upload-files/gorimpmod-rmwsegintheor_r5_web_0.pdf.

21. This section is adapted from Practice Greenhealth, "University of Minnesota Medical Center, Fairview: OR Kit Reformulation," Greening the OR Case Study, https://practicegreenhealth.org/sites/default/files/upload-files/casestudy_uofmn_r5_web.pdf.

22. Kevin Hoyde, "Greening the OR: OR Kit Reformulation," Practice Greenhealth Webinar, October 18, 2011.

23. Kaiser Permanente, "Reducing Operating Room Waste with Sterile Wrap Recycling," April 2010, https://practicegreenhealth.org/sites/default/files/upload-files/sterile_wrap_recycling_success_story_4.10.pdf.

24. Freedonia, "Disposable Medical Supplies to 2016—Demand and Sales Forecasts, Market Share, Market Size, Market Leaders," Study no. 2853 (March 2012), http://www.freedoniagroup.com/Disposable-Medical-Supplies.html.

25. US GAO, "Reprocessed Single-Use Medical Devices: FDA Oversight Has Increased, and Available Information Does Not Indicate That Use Presents an Elevated Health Risk" (January 2008), http://www.gao.gov/new.items/d08147.pdf.

26. Practice Greenhealth and Greening the OR, "Implementation Module: Medical Device Reprocessing," https://practicegreenhealth.org/sites/default/files/upload-files/gorimpmod-meddevicerepr_r5_web.pdf.

27. US FDA, "Executive Summary: Survey on the Reuse and Reprocessing of Single-Use Devices (SUDs) in US Hospitals," April 30, 2009, http://www.fda.gov/MedicalDevices/DeviceRegulationandGuidance/ReprocessingofSingle-UseDevices/ucm121678.htm.

28. Practice Greenhealth, "Metro Health Hospital, Wyoming, MI: Medical Device Reprocessing," Practice Greenhealth Case Study, https://practicegreenhealth.org/sites/default/files/upload-files/casestudy_metrohealth_r4_web.pdf, and Practice Greenhealth, "Greening the OR: Guidance Documents," http://www.c4spgh.org/HCW1_Presentations/GOR_FullSet_Guidance%20Docs_Web_042711.pdf.

29. Practice Greenehalth, "Greening the OR: Guidance Documents."

30. Practice Greenhealth, *2012 Sustainability Benchmark Report* (August 2012).

31. "Kaiser Permanente Turns Green," press release, April 18, 2003; see also Kaiser Permanente, "An Earth Day Round Up of Kaiser Permanent's Recent Environmental Stewardship Work," http://share.kaiserpermanente.org/article/an-earth-day-round-up-of-kaiser-permanentes-recent-environmental-stewardship-work/.

32. Tieszen and Gruenberg, "A Quantitative, Qualitative and Critical Assessment of Surgical Waste."

33. Nancy Jenkins, "How to Reduce Waste by Increasing Use of Reusable Medical Textiles," *Supply Chain Strategies and Solutions* 6, no. 2 (2011), http://www.arta1.com/cms/uploads/How_to_Reduce_Waste_NJenkins.pdf.

34. John Ebers, moderator, "Reusable Surgical Textiles: A Means to Save Money and Reduce OR Waste Up to 30 Percent," Greening the OR webinar, February 17, 2011.

35. T. Grimmond et al., "Sharps Injury Reduction Using Sharpsmart™," *Journal of Hospital Infection* 54, no. 3 (2003): 232–238.

36. AASHE, "Harvard Medical School Reusable Sharps Container Pilot," http://www.aashe.org/resources/case-studies/harvard-medical-school-reusable-sharps-container-pilot. Also, Practice Greenhealth has a webinar that can be purchased: www.practicegreenhealth.org

37. Ano Lobb, "Sustainable Health IT: A Plan for Healthcare-Generated e-Waste?" *JustMeans* (blog), April 19, 2011, http://www.justmeans.com/blogs/sustainable-health-it-a-plan-for-healthcare-generated-e-waste.

38. Elizabeth Dwoskin "Keeping Conflict Minerals out of Your Cell Phone," *Bloomberg BusinessWeek,* April 12, 2012, http://www.businessweek.com/articles/2012-04-12/keeping-conflict-minerals-out-of-your-cell-phone.

39. US SEC, "SEC Adopts Rule for Disclosing Use of Conflict Minerals," press release, http://www.sec.gov/news/press/2012/2012-163.htm.

40. California Integrated Waste Management Board, *California 2008 Statewide Waste Characterization Study* (Sacramento: Integrated Waste Management Board, 2009), http://www.calrecycle.ca.gov/Publications/Detail.aspx?PublicationID=1346.

41. This section is from Practice Greenhealth, "All from Greening: The OR Case Study," 2011, and "Winner's Circle," *Greenhealth* (2012), http://greenhealthmagazine.org/winners-circle/.

42. Oregon Sustainable Hospitals Roundtable, case study, Providence Health System, November 2009. See also Andre Meunier, "It's a Recyclable Picnic for 3,000, as St. Vincent's Throws Barbecue—and Leaves 1 Bin of Trash," *The Oregonian,* June 18, 2009.

6

Green Chemicals and the Detoxing of Health Care

M ounting concern about the health impacts of chemicals in health care and in daily life is mostly a modern-day phenomenon, stemming largely from the explosion in the development of synthetic industrial chemicals over the past half-century. During this period, tens of thousands of new synthetic chemicals have been developed and have found their way into every niche and corner of the consumer society. But scientific efforts to understand the health impacts of our chemically saturated environment, and government efforts to enforce some safety standards over that environment, is an older story, and one that may shed some interesting light on our current concerns.

The first published scientific report linking a chemical compound commonly found in the environment to a chronic illness was published in the year 1775 by an eminent London surgeon, Sir Purcival Pott. Among his many accomplishments, Sir Purcival established that a type of cancer of the scrotum that was common among London chimney sweeps in their thirties and forties was linked to their exposure to chimney soot— not as adults, but as young children. The victims had been apprenticed as pauper children to adult master chimney sweeps at ages as young as 4 or 5 years, and they had been literally stuffed up and down London's peculiarly angular and narrow chimneys for most of their prepubescent lives. Pott's study probably led to the same sort of headlines that follow similarly sensational scientific reports today, for 13 years later Parliament finally responded by passing the Chimney Sweepers Act to protect child labor. The first version of the act stipulated that no child could serve as an apprentice chimney sweep under the age of 8 and children had to be provided suitable clothing, allowed to attend church, and be given a bath at least once a week.[1]

What is interesting about the chimney sweeps cancer story is not just the Dickensian horror of it, but the parallels to our own efforts to understand and respond appropriately to chemical hazards. Subsequent research on coal soot in the nineteenth century showed that the actual compound responsible for the later-life cancers among the London chimney sweeps was benzo(a)pyrene, a mutagenic and carcinogenic aromatic hydrocarbon that even today remains a serious health hazard as a component of tobacco smoke.[2]

CHEMICALS AND HEALTH:
THE DARK SIDE OF THE MIRACLE

Barely a week passes without yet another disturbing report in the headlines linking some common consumer product or industrial process to cancers, Alzheimer's disease, Parkinson's disease, autoimmune disorders, neurological conditions, depression, or any number of other chronic disorders that account for many of the twenty-first century's health problems and health care costs. The culprits, most often, are not the products or the processes, per se, but hazards lurking within the molecular composition of their constituent parts—the chemicals that have made the last half-century both a marvel of improved human health and progress and a dangerous, mostly unexplored minefield of toxic timebombs.

A growing body of scientific literature suggests, with increasing confidence, that some significant share of the 84,000 industrial chemicals registered for use in the Toxic Substances Control Act's chemical inventory,[3] plus the thousand or more new compounds added to it annually, are among the key environmental determinants of chronic diseases that today affect an estimated 133 million Americans.[4] They include a vast variety of synthetic chemicals, metals, compounds, and related elements that are now ubiquitous in the world's food, water, soil, air, buildings, and even in our own bodies. We use them to make pesticides, industrial solvents, personal care products, pharmaceuticals, cleansers, food products and food containers, furniture, sealants, paint, and paint removers—literally millions of items we rely on every day. In fact, some 97 percent of all the goods bought and sold in the United States incorporate synthetic chemicals of one sort or another.[5] While estimates of the disease burden attributable to chemicals are imprecise, the World Health Organization conservatively estimates that chemicals are responsible for roughly 8 percent of all disease worldwide.[6] In the United States, researchers estimate that chemicals may be responsible for 5 percent of childhood cancers and as much as 30 percent of childhood asthma.[7] It has been estimated that exposures of children age 5 and under to the chemicals in household cleaning products alone are responsible for as many as 12,000 visits to US hospital emergency rooms annually.[8]

Chemicals in Health Care

Ironically, the health care sector, with its commitment to "do no harm," is a large user of chemicals, spending more than $100 billion a year on chemicals and chemical products annually (excluding pharmaceuticals).[9] Adding to the irony, these chemicals include a host of products used to treat us when we are ill and to maintain a clean and safe environment for patients and staff at all times—cleaners and disinfectants; flame retardants and formaldehyde in furniture; chemicals of concern inside medical devices, like IV bags and tubing; solvents and formaldehyde in laboratories; noxious emissions from anesthetic gases; prescription antidepressants, anticonvulsants, steroids, chemotherapy drugs, antibiotics, and other biologically powerful medications that, improperly disposed of, end up in our drinking water. They include chemicals with known or suspected life-cycle impacts, capable of harming patients, health care workers, and communities from the day they are manufactured until decades after their disposal.

As mentioned in Chapter 1, I decided, in 2005, to take my research on chemicals and toxins from the statistical to the personal level. I was already familiar with the Centers for Disease Control and Prevention's (CDC) National Biomonitoring Program, which periodically tests the blood and urine of several hundred Americans for the presence of more than 200 high-production chemicals.[10] I wondered about my own level of exposure, and so I agreed to be part of a small cohort tested for the presence of just 27 common industrial chemicals.

When the results came in, I learned that I had measureable amounts of all 27 chemicals, including mercury, flame retardants, bisphenol A (BPA), pesticides (including DDT, which was banned in 1972 but lingers in the environment), perfluorochemicals, and phthalates. Dr. Michael McCally, an eminent public health physician and environmental health scientist who was the physician of record for the study, explained that my results were, unfortunately, typical.

A few years later, Physicians for Social Responsibility (PSR), a medical and public health group known for its work on nuclear weapons, climate change, and environmental toxins, in partnership with the American Nurses Association and Health Care Without Harm, conducted its own biomonitoring investigation. It focused on the exposure of health care providers to six chemicals or chemical groups (62 in all) that are believed to be associated with certain diseases and that are widely used in health care settings. Sadly, it confirmed just how typical I was. The study, which examined physicians and nurses from across the nation, found that every participant had at least 24 individual chemicals present, 18 of which were present in all participants. Virtually everyone had detectable levels of BPA, phthalates, polybrominated diphenylethers (PBDEs) used in flame retardants, and perfluorochemicals (PFCs), all of which have been associated with chronic illnesses, including various cancers and endocrine malfunction.[11]

Dr. George Lundgren, a family practice physician from Minneapolis and a study participant, commented upon learning his results, "When you do find out some of the specific unnatural chemicals in your body it is hard to deny, minimize, rationalize, or justify their presence. It is disturbing to know the only body I have is permanently contaminated."

I know the feeling.

Health Impacts: What We Know and What We Do Not Know

We literally live and work in a chemical soup, and we know far more about its many benefits than about its potential hazards. Apart from a handful of substances that have been thoroughly studied, tested, and determined to be harmful, such as lead, mercury, some pesticides, and arsenic, the vast majority of the more than 3,000 chemicals in high-volume production (1 million pounds per year) today have not been tested for toxicity or their impact on human health or the environment.[12] This is due in part to ineffective laws, overlapping jurisdictions among agencies, underfunding for research on environmental health determinants, and other factors. As the late Senator Frank Lautenberg said in 2009: "Far too little is known about the hundreds of chemicals that end up in our bodies, and the US Environmental Protection Agency (EPA) has far too little authority to deal with the chemicals that science has already proven dangerous."[13] To which the President's Cancer Panel, after investigating the state of knowledge on environmental carcinogens in 2010, added: "We know enough to act."[14]

In fact, despite our paucity of knowledge about the health effects of most specific chemicals and mixtures of chemicals, the modern sciences involved in research on chemical safety and toxicology have progressed considerably in recent decades. We now know, for instance, that the old axiom that "the dose makes the poison," which served as the basis for classical toxicology, is at best only half true. High doses of almost any substance can be toxic, but that does not mean, as it was long assumed, that there is a lower dose level at which the same substance is safe.

Lead, for instance, cannot be safely ingested at any dose level, nor can asbestos.[15]

Additionally, we now know that certain pollutants are extremely persistent and accumulate in living organisms, undergoing a process known as biomagnification as they move from one organism to another up the food chain, growing ever more concentrated and hazardous along the way. At any point in one's life, even low-level exposures to certain chemicals can result in significant health problems, if not tomorrow perhaps a decade or more later—or even a generation later.

We also have learned that chemicals can have opposing or synergistic effects on one another, making some combinations of chemicals even more toxic than the individual chemicals alone. Tobacco smoke, for instance, is a well-established carcinogen, but when a cigarette smoker is also exposed to asbestos, another carcinogen, the risk of lung cancer can be increased by 50 to 84 times.[16]

And finally, we are learning that many hazardous and toxic chemicals do not stop being hazardous at the end of their useful life when they are deposited in hazardous waste sites, 70 percent of which have breached their containment and leaked their contents into soil and/or groundwater. The US EPA expects to require 217,000 new hazardous waste sites nationwide by 2033 for the cleanup of as many as 350,000 contaminated industrial sites.[17]

Infants at Greatest Risk

Modern science has confirmed another important lesson about chemicals and health: the fact that children are not merely "little adults." This was one of the most important lessons established by the National Research Council's (NRC) 1993 report *Pesticides in the Diets of Infants and Children*, which led to a sea change in the way health risks from chemicals and other potentially toxic substances are studied and assessed.[18] Prior to this report, the government's regulatory system for assessing the health risks of pesticides did not consider—and researchers did not study—the unique physiological characteristics of children, infants, or fetuses; substances were assessed for risks only to the "average adult."[19]

As the NRC report notes, there are vast differences between children and adults when it comes to their susceptibility to chemicals and pesticides. For instance, children's intake of food, water, and air per pound of body weight is several orders of magnitude greater than that of adults. Children's sensitivity to exposure of toxic substances is similarly greater than that of adults. Also, due to their underdeveloped metabolic pathways, children's ability to metabolize toxins is poor compared to that of adults. And finally, the report noted that "compared to late-in-life exposures, exposures... early in life can lead to a greater risk of chronic effects that are expressed only after long latency periods have elapsed."[20] During an infant's prenatal life and the first few years following birth, the complex development of critical organs, like the brain and the reproductive system, can easily be disrupted by exposure to toxins that would have no impact on an adult.[21]

We have little knowledge of the full extent to which fetuses and developing newborns are exposed to toxic chemicals via placental blood, but early research provides cause for concern. A 2005 study by the Environmental Working Group found an average of 200 industrial chemicals and pollutants in the umbilical cord blood from 10 randomly selected infants born over a 2-month period to volunteer mothers in the Red Cross's national cord blood collection program.[22] None of the mothers worked in the chemical industry or were known to have suffered from chemical exposures. A total of 287 chemicals were detected throughout the cohort, including eight perfluorochemicals (used as stain and oil repellants in fast food packaging, clothes, and textiles); dozens of widely used brominated flame retardants and their toxic by-products; and numerous pesticides. At least 180 of the detected chemicals were known or suspected to be related to cancer in humans or animals, and 208 were related to birth defects or abnormal development in animal studies.

The rapidly expanding knowledge about the complex ways that chemicals can impact human health, especially in infants and children, has produced a surge of peer-reviewed studies pointing to potential links between environmental chemicals and the increasing rates of childhood asthma (the leading cause of pediatric hospitalization), birth defects (the leading cause of infant death), and neurodevelopmental disorders like dyslexia, mental retardation, autism, attention-deficit disorder, and other learning disabilities.[23] Recent research has added obesity to the list of chronic disorders that can be triggered in later life by exposure to endocrine-disrupting chemicals in the womb or during early childhood. These so-called obesogens include such common chemicals as DES; BPA; PFCs used in clothing, furniture, carpets, packaging, and cookware; and some phthalates.[24]

DES, which used to be prescribed to pregnant women to prevent miscarriage and other complications of pregnancy, was mostly discontinued in 1971 after it was found to be related to an increased risk of a once rare vaginal and cervical cancer in young women who were exposed in utero to DES. Further research found that women who took DES while pregnant have a higher rate of breast cancer and that their daughters also are at greater risk of infertility, reproductive tract structural changes, and pregnancy complications. Now, researchers are finding evidence of a higher risk of cancer and birth defects among the *granddaughters* of DES women—two generations removed from the initial exposure.[25]

Bisphenol A: Today's Poster Hazard

Today's most controversial endocrine disrupter may be BPA, which since the early 1960s has been widely used, with approval of the Food and Drug Administration, in a vast variety of products containing plastics and epoxy resins. BPA has been used in some medical equipment, such as dental sealants and machines used for cardiopulmonary bypass operations and dialysis procedures. It has also been a component in baby bottles, sippy cups, and in food and beverage cans from which the chemical can leach into people's daily diet. In 2003, the CDC's biomonitoring program found detectable levels of the substance in 93 percent of the more than 2,500 urine samples from people 6 years and older.[26]

The FDA has long maintained that BPA is safe, based on studies that show levels of the substance used in commercial products are not toxic—meaning they would not harm humans. But since the late 1990s, a growing body of research by endocrinologists, molecular biologists, reproductive specialists, and others has raised concerns that even the low levels of BPA that leach from consumer or medical products can cause cellular changes that may contribute to obesity; diabetes; reproductive disorders; prostate, breast, and uterine cancer; asthma; and cardiovascular disease.[27] Kaiser Permanente's Division of Research published four studies linking BPA to decreased sexual function in men, decreased sperm concentration and vitality, and low birth weight in infants born to women exposed to BPA in the workplace.[28] Both animal and human studies have shown that BPA can pass through the placental barrier and that fetuses are likely to be exposed to similar (if not higher) levels of BPA as those of their mothers.[29]

Such findings have prompted Canada, China, Malaysia, Turkey, much of Europe, and 11 US states to ban the use of BPA in baby bottles, as of 2012. Every major baby bottle manufacturer and packager of infant formula ceased using the chemical as a result of strenuous consumer pressure and lobbying by the Breast Cancer Fund's Cans Not Cancer campaign and other health advocacy groups. Yet the FDA continued to uphold its approval of BPA for infant formula containers until July 2012, when it finally bent to pressure from—of all places—the American Chemistry Council, the chemical industry trade group. The council was concerned about consumer confusion over conflicting regulations, not to mention plummeting confidence in its members' products.[30] And even then, the FDA ban did not apply to BPA in other containers, such as food cans or baby food jar lids.

Health Care Bears the Burden of Response

For those of us who work in health care, whether we are care providers or administrators, what is most disturbing about the outpouring of new knowledge on chemical toxicity is the fear that the science is fast outpacing the ability of many in the health care sector to respond to it. And we are getting little help from federal regulators. The burden of absorbing the science and acting on it has been left to doctors, nurses, and managers who have little or no training in toxicology, despite their expertise in medicine and their devotion to their patients.

I am reminded, once again, of the dismay registered by that caring neonatal nurse at our San Francisco medical center, discussed in Chapter 1, on learning that so many of the PVC-based medical devices used to treat ill newborns could be leaching a toxic substance into their bodies. Fortunately, as a large, highly integrated health care system, we were able to act by running our own series of clinical trials to identify PVC- and DEHP-free alternatives to devices used in the most intensive procedures and by persuading our equipment supplier to seek out additional alternative products. By early 2012, we were able to convert virtually all of our IV medical equipment, including more than 9 million solution bags to PVC- and DEHP-free alternatives, and 5 million tubing sets to DEHP-free products. But in the absence of clear and consistent regulatory policies, many health systems continue to struggle with the knowledge that much of the equipment and products used throughout hospitals and clinics to save lives and safeguard against health hazards is itself hazardous.

TURNING THE TIDE ON TOXICS

Understanding and acting on the risks of chemical exposures in health care are daunting tasks for which there are few examples of comprehensive solutions. Furthermore, few health care organizations have the staff expertise to grapple with the bewildering array of the thousands of potentially harmful chemicals that are used in the manufacture of common, everyday cleaning products, building materials, industrial solvents, disinfectants, and a multitude of other products used throughout health care facilities. The fact is, most chemists do not study toxicology themselves and do not know much more about the toxic potentials of the cleaning products they produce than do the maintenance people who use them, and often suffer from them, to keep hospitals clean and sanitary.

Getting Started

Lack of expertise about toxins need not be an excuse for lack of action by health care systems. Experts at Health Care Without Harm, Practice Greenhealth, and Physicians for Social Responsibility, among others, have produced a wealth of online information about sustainability issues in health care, including helpful information and tools about potentially harmful chemicals. As more hospitals and health systems act on this information to develop comprehensive chemicals policies, we are already beginning to see fundamental changes in the design, manufacture, use, transparency, regulation, and disposal of chemicals, all driving toward improved human and ecosystem health.

Health Care Without Harm's publication "A Guide to Choosing Safer Products and Chemicals: Implementing Chemicals Policy in Health Care" is a great place to start for health systems large or small. Available online through the organization's website at http://www.noharm.org, it covers actions that organizations need to take both internally and externally, including engaging with product vendors and advocating for policy change at the state and federal levels.

INTERNAL ACTIONS

Internally, the first step on the road to safer chemicals is making an institutional commitment, fully supported by senior leadership, in the form of a simple statement of the organization's broad goals and principles. Kaiser Permanente's safer chemicals statement begins with a clear declaration that "Kaiser Permanente commits to advancing an economy where chemicals used in commerce are not harmful to humans or the environment." It then aligns that aspiration with the organization's social mission and its environmental stewardship vision, as well as two important environmental principles:

- The Precautionary Principle: Where there is credible evidence that a material we are using may result in environmental or public health harm, we should strive to replace it with safer alternatives that meet our performance criteria.[31]

- The Extended Producer Responsibility (EPR) Principle: A producer's responsibility for a product extends to the postconsumer stage of the product's life cycle. This means that chemical and product manufacturers have a responsibility for the health impacts of the chemicals they use and the products they create. It also means that purchasers of those products and chemicals have the right to request safety testing and full disclosure of the results. This provides incentives to producers to take environmental considerations into account in the design of their products.[32]

The next step is to define exactly what actions the organization is willing to commit to in terms of managing chemicals in their operations. The Business NGO Working Group, representing several dozen businesses and environmental groups promoting safer chemicals and sustainable materials, has defined the following guiding principles, each of which has been endorsed and adopted by leading health systems, including Kaiser Permanente and Dignity Health, as well as major health care product purchasing organizations, like Novation and Premier, Inc.:

- **Understand product chemistry**: To even begin moving toward safer products, organizations need to know what chemicals are contained in the products they are purchasing, information that only the product manufacturers and chemical suppliers can provide. How does an organization access this information? By requesting it—and then acting on it through health care's purchasing power.
- **Assess and avoid hazards:** Again, this important step requires organizations with purchasing muscle to flex it. Doing so, we can encourage product suppliers to use chemicals in their products that have low or no hazard potential and to eliminate chemicals of high concern (meaning chemicals known or suspected of being persistent, bioaccumulative, and toxic, as well as any that are carcinogenic, mutagenic, or endocrine disruptors). When hazards cannot be prevented, exposure to products should be minimized.

A useful resource for quick access to reliable information on products' chemical characteristics, alternative products, and undesirable materials is the list of databases compiled by the Toxics Use Reduction Institute at the University of Massachusetts at Lowell, which is online at http://www.turi.org.

- **Commit to continuous improvement:** Organizations need to create internal governance structures and policies for the regular review of product and process chemistry and that promote the use of chemicals, processes, and products with inherently lower hazard potentials.

- **Support public policies and industry standards** that advance the implementation of the first three principles, eliminate or reduce known hazards, and promote a greener economy, including support for green chemistry research and education.

In addition to these steps, a good organizational chemicals policy should prioritize workplace safety for health care providers and other staff, including maintenance workers who routinely handle potentially hazardous cleaning materials. Every facility should have at least one staff committee charged with developing and overseeing an occupational safety program that focuses on decreasing chemical exposures. (Note that this is a job for which nurses are particularly interested and adept.)

To facilitate implementation of the aforementioned four principles, in 2012 BizNGO released the comprehensive "Guide to Safer Chemicals," which is useful for setting benchmarks for how manufacturers, retailers, and purchasers can track their progress on using chemicals in products that are safer for human and environmental health.

External Actions: Flexing Your Purchasing Muscle

Executing a product purchasing policy is one way health care organizations can exert their greatest strength in pursuit of a safer chemicals regimen. After all, the health care sector is one of the biggest purchasers of a variety of chemically laden products, such as exam gloves, plastic tubing, cleaning products, and disinfectants.

In the beginning stages of implementing an environmental preferable purchasing (EPP) policy, it is important to alert current vendors before implementing new contract requirements. This can be done with a standard statement of intent or request for proposal (RFP) stipulating that, as of a certain date, your organization intends to deal only with suppliers willing to provide specific information about products and willing to identify acceptable alternative products if necessary. It is useful, as well, to identify subsets of targeted chemical products that represent the greatest hazards to the greatest number of patients, staff, and the surrounding community. These products may differ from one organization to another.

Health care organizations should create a target list of types of chemicals that represent the greatest hazards for their operations. Practice Greenhealth offers a comprehensive list of resources and tools for implementing EPP policies, including standard request for proposal language, guides to green products, case studies of EPPs in action, EPP consulting services, and standardized environmental questions to include in requests for proposals for medical products.

Kaiser Permanente has developed a supplier disclosure scorecard (see Chapter 7 on purchasing strategies) that is used for purchasing medical products across the entire system. It requires suppliers to disclose if the products they are bidding to us contain the following types of chemicals:

- Persistent, bioaccumulative, and toxic chemicals, known as PBTs.
- Carcinogens and reproductive toxicants listed by California's Proposition 65 list of chemicals that cause cancer or reproductive harm.
- Halogenated flame retardants.
- Phthalates (including DEHP), polyvinyl chloride, BPA, latex, and mercury.

Using this process, we have been able to identify a number of safer alternatives to potentially harmful products or, in some cases, prompt the development of safer alternatives. And in many cases, because we are a very large purchaser, we have been able to effect major changes across entire product lines, thereby benefiting the entire health care sector. I discuss this further in Chapter 7.

A good example of the power of purchasing is our experience in moving away from powdered latex and polyvinyl chloride exam gloves. Back in the late 1990s, a number of studies reported that significant percentages of individuals, particularly doctors, nurses, and other health care workers, were allergic or sensitive to latex. Vinyl gloves, meanwhile, create dioxin pollution as a by-product of both manufacturing and disposal. We mounted an aggressive effort, led by a dermatologist, to identify high-quality alternatives to latex and vinyl, and finally decided to purchase gloves made of nitrile. That decision affected the entire medical glove industry, because we used more than 50 million gloves annually. Within a few years, more manufacturers changed their product line to include vinyl-free, latex-safe materials, and the increased supply brought the costs down. Today we use more than 300 million vinyl-free and latex-safe gloves a year.

Similarly, in 2002 we put out a challenge to the market to create a greener, PVC-free carpet suitable for health care facilities that did not exist at the time. Within 14 months, Tandus, our existing carpet supplier, developed a carpet with backing made from the film that's left over from recycled laminated safety (windshield) glass. By 2004, the new product was on the market. Since then, some 10 million square feet of PVC-free carpet has been installed in our facilities at a cost equivalent to the old contract. We have realized similar successes in our campaign to become PVC-free and DEHP-free with purchases of other medical products and materials, including neonatal IV systems, reflective roofing, flooring, fabric, and bumper and corner guards throughout the hallways of our medical facilities.

In 2009, we adopted a new, multiyear safer chemicals strategy that involved performing detailed chemical hazard assessments on a broad range of products that ultimately generated our "Targeted Ten" list of products. This is a list of things pervasive in our facilities that could expose patients and staff to chemicals of concern, as defined in our Environmentally Preferable Purchasing policy. The list included IV tubing and solution bags, dialysis tubing, high-level disinfectants, fixatives, solvents, enzymatic detergents, janitorial cleaning chemicals, cabinetry and casework, paint, and resilient flooring. We made a commitment to contract for safer alternatives by 2013, wherever we could find alternatives that met all clinical and performance requirements.

Our purchase of Green Seal–certified general-purpose cleaners increased from 34 percent to 79 percent of our overall spending on cleaning products, excluding floor care products, for which we could not find a suitable set of products in our first round of testing. To strengthen the move to safer cleaning products, we also concluded a contract with our external janitorial service providers obligating them to use only products specified by Kaiser Permanente. In the area of high-level disinfectants, we converted 30 percent of all products, totaling 100,000 liters annually, to a peroxide-based disinfectant that eliminates skin and respiratory sensitization among patients and staff. That conversion had the added benefit of increasing efficiency by decreasing the time it takes to disinfect endoscopes and probes by 40 percent.

None of this is easy. Identifying chemicals of high concern in products and identifying and evaluating safer alternatives that meet health care's demanding performance standards at affordable costs can require years or even decades of investment in staff time and expertise, which is simply not feasible for most organizations. As I told a congressional committee a few years ago when I testified regarding the Toxic Substances Control Act, when we went in search of alternatives to PVC flooring, we had to invent our own testing protocol and use in-house, certified industrial hygienists to perform tests in order to understand the health implications of the alternatives.[33] How many organizations can do that? And sometimes, the alternatives we have identified have later been shown to have their own health risks.

Despite the great strides that we and other large systems have achieved through our purchasing muscle, we still experience limitations in achieving our goal of using products and materials that are environmentally sustainable and safe for our patients and staff. We have come to recognize that, while the health care sector can play a leadership role in turning the tide against toxic or unsafe products, what is really needed to take safety and sustainability to a new level are transformative and closely related changes in two sectors outside of health care: the chemical and chemical product manufacturing industries, and the regulatory agencies that oversee those industries.

GREEN CHEMISTRY

The first of these requirements, a safe and sustainable chemical products manufacturing sector, may take a generation or more to develop into maturity. But the early seeds are already sprouting thanks to a nascent movement known as "green chemistry." The movement dates back to the 1990 Pollution Prevention Act, when the US EPA began funding research projects aimed at carrying out the law's declared policy that "pollution should be prevented or reduced at the source, whenever feasible," rather than just cleaned up afterward.[34]

The US EPA defines green chemistry, also known as sustainable chemistry, as "the design of chemical products and processes that reduce or eliminate the use or generation of hazardous substances."[35] The discipline, it adds, "applies across the life cycle of a chemical product, including its design, manufacture, and use," all the way to its disposal as waste (see Box 6.1).

Box 6.1 THE TWELVE PRINCIPLES OF GREEN CHEMISTRY

Paul Anastas, who coined the term "green chemistry" in 1991 when he was at the US EPA, and John C. Warner developed twelve principles of green chemistry, which are widely recognized by advocates of the discipline.

1. **Prevention.** It is better to prevent waste than to treat or clean up waste after it has been created.
2. **Atom economy.** Synthetic methods should be designed to maximize the incorporation of all materials used in the process into the final product.
3. **Less hazardous chemical syntheses.** Wherever practicable, synthetic methods should be designed to use and generate

substances that possess little or no toxicity to human health and the environment.

4. **Designing safer chemicals.** Chemical products should be designed to affect their desired function while minimizing their toxicity.

5. **Safer solvents and auxiliaries.** The use of auxiliary substances (e.g., solvents, separation agents, etc.) should be made unnecessary wherever possible and innocuous when used.

6. **Design for energy efficiency.** Energy requirements of chemical processes should be recognized for their environmental and economic impacts and should be minimized. If possible, synthetic methods should be conducted at ambient temperature and pressure.

7. **Use of renewable feedstocks.** A raw material or feedstock should be renewable rather than depleting whenever technically and economically practicable.

8. **Reduce derivatives.** Unnecessary derivatization (use of blocking groups, protection/ deprotection, temporary modification of physical/chemical processes) should be minimized or avoided if possible, because such steps require additional reagents and can generate waste.

9. **Catalysis.** Catalytic reagents (as selective as possible) are superior to stoichiometric reagents.

10. **Design for degradation.** Chemical products should be designed so that at the end of their function they break down into innocuous degradation products and do not persist in the environment.

11. **Real-time analysis for pollution prevention.** Analytical methodologies need to be further developed to allow for real-time, in-process monitoring and control prior to the formation of hazardous substances.

12. **Inherently safer chemistry for accident prevention.** Substances and the form of a substance used in a chemical process should be chosen to minimize the potential for chemical accidents, including releases, explosions, and fires.[36]

Over the past two decades, the US EPA's own Green Chemistry Program has helped spark growing interest and activity in the design and manufacture of environmentally sustainable chemicals and chemical processes in major academic centers, among a handful of state governments, and among a growing number of major chemical product manufacturers. A report in 2011 by the clean technology market research firm Navigant Research estimated that the market for green chemistry products could grow from $2.8 billion in 2011 to nearly $100 billion within a decade, driven by the need for renewable, bio-based feedstocks for production of chemicals.[37] As impressive as that sounds, the report notes that the projected green chemistry market would still represent a small fraction of the global chemical industry, which is expected to grow to $5.3 trillion (with a "t") in the same period.

A good example of the kinds of products now emerging from green chemistry research comes from one of the annual award winners of the US EPA's Presidential Green Chemistry Challenge. In 2012, Geoffrey W. Coates, of Cornell University, was recognized for developing an innovative process to synthesize plastics, which normally are derived from fossil fuels, from inexpensive, bio-renewable substances, including carbon dioxide, carbon monoxide, plant oils, and lactic acid. The process has already been used by a commercial start-up to develop industrial coil coatings, and it may prove useful in developing coatings to replace the BPA resins used in the coatings that line food and drink cans.

A similar project, known as the Bio-Plastics Pilot, involves a partnership among Health Care Without Harm, a prominent green chemistry research lab, and a bio-based startup company to develop a variety of bio-based polymers for use in durable and semidurable health care products.[38]

On the academic front, a number of major universities, including Yale University, the University of Massachusetts, Carnegie Mellon, the University of Oregon, and the University of California at Berkeley, have launched degree programs in green chemistry. UC Berkeley sponsors The Berkeley Center for Green Chemistry, for instance, which seeks nothing less than "a generational transformation in society's production and use of chemicals and materials."[39] It is an interdisciplinary program in Berkeley's colleges of chemistry, public health, engineering, natural resources, law, and the Haas business school. Its lofty mission is threefold: to train a new generation of chemists committed to safety and sustainability, to conduct research on safe chemicals, and to make the best available science on chemistry and toxicology transparent for policymakers, manufacturers, and the public. As the Center's former associate director, Michael Wilson argued in a recent speech, green chemistry is really about saving the US chemical industry from itself: "By embracing the science and technology of green chemistry, our nation can retain a robust domestic industrial chemical industry that will be capable of responding to the growing global demand for safer chemistries not with denial and rhetoric in the face of declining market share, but with global leadership in innovation, in accountability, and proactive action."[40]

Major ongoing research at the center provides a glimpse of the kinds of impacts green chemistry could have, not only in health care but across the entire economy. One key research area is addressing chemical challenges in the greater use of biomass materials as renewable sources of hydrocarbons to produce clean, affordable energy and reduce greenhouse gas emissions. Another project is focused on developing new chemical tests for screening large numbers of chemicals and chemical mixtures as possible contributors to breast cancer. Other projects are working on development of nontoxic dispersants for use in marine oil spills and compilation of a public, online database, known as the Public Library of Materials (PLUM), detailing authoritative information about the known health hazards of thousands of chemicals.

GREENING PUBLIC POLICY AT THE STATE LEVEL
Besides the maturing of a green chemistry market, the other requirement for a decisive turn toward sustainable product manufacturing is the strengthening of the regulatory system that governs chemicals. Today, in the absence of strong federal regulation, California and several other states have led the way in creating policies aimed at protecting the public from the health and environmental hazards of known or suspected chemicals and other toxic materials.

One example of how difficult it is to change state policy is the 38-year controversy over flame retardants in California. In November 2013, Governor Brown approved a new flame retardant standard that revises a law he approved in his first term as governor in 1975. The original standard (Technical Bulletin 117) required furniture manufacturers to use several pounds of toxic chemicals in each piece of upholstered furniture for sale in California. Quite the opposite of protecting the health of Californians, the standard resulted in the use of massive quantities of toxic chemicals by the furniture industry, chemicals that are now detected in the bodies of virtually all Americans. The new standard, aptly named Technical Bulletin 117-2013, took effect January 1, 2014, and does not ban flame retardants, but rather it establishes a new test that furniture makers can meet without using toxic chemicals.

California's experience with trying to regulate hazardous substances is indicative of both the possibilities and the problems encountered at the local or state level. As early as 1986, California passed Proposition 65, a voter-approved initiative to reduce or eliminate exposures to toxic materials that cause cancer, birth defects, or other reproductive harm. The law works in two ways: by prohibiting businesses from knowingly discharging listed substances into drinking water sources, including land sources, and by prohibiting the known exposure of individuals to listed substances (now numbering more than 800) without providing a "clear and reasonable" warning. The warning can be given by a variety of means, including printed product labels, signs posted at buildings, or notices published in a newspaper. However, the warnings only indicate that something in the product or building may cause cancer or affect reproduction; it does not indicate what the substance is, how someone might be exposed to it, or how to reduce exposure.

Proposition 65 remains highly controversial in California, but both sides of the ongoing debate acknowledge it has had major impacts in reduction of exposures to hazardous substances and in encouraging product manufacturers to reformulate their products rather than list them. An analysis of air emissions of all toxic chemicals in Proposition 65–listed products, comparing California emissions to nationwide emissions, found that 10 years after implementation of the law, concentrations of those chemicals had fallen to just 10 percent of the 1988 base year, while US levels remained at about 35 percent of the base year.[41]

In 2008, more comprehensive legislation, known as the Green Chemistry Initiative, was signed into law with the aim of regulating the creation and use of existing materials deemed hazardous to the environment and human health. It seeks to promote a "preventive medicine" approach to new chemicals at the design and manufacturing stages, making good on the 1990 federal Pollution Prevention Act's goal of source prevention as opposed to mitigation. The legislation created a blue-ribbon science panel to promote research, set up an online database on toxins, and drew up proposed regulations for assessing alternatives to hazardous products. Ideally, the law sought to use a regulatory framework to spark investment and innovation in the science and technology of safer chemicals.

Unfortunately, the law ran into a strong headwind of stakeholder objections that it was either too lenient or too stringent. After 4 years of delayed implementation, final regulations were issued in mid-2012, with endorsements by Kaiser Permanente and other health care organizations and advocacy groups.

In addition to the California initiative, Connecticut, Maine, Michigan, Minnesota, and Washington have also passed green chemistry legislation or enacted executive orders to reduce the use of toxic chemicals, prioritize harmful chemicals, and identify safer alternatives.[42] At least a half dozen other states are considering such legislation.

REFORMING NATIONAL CHEMICAL POLICY: THE TOXIC SUBSTANCES CONTROL ACT

Despite some progress at the state level, few advocates for chemical reform believe that a patchwork of inconsistent regulations and rules across the country is ideal for either the goal of human and environmental health or the economic health of product manufacturers and retailers. As California EPA Secretary Linda Adams said in response to her state's Green Chemistry Initiative, "In the absence of a unifying approach, interest groups and policy makers have been attempting to take these issues on one-by-one. We need a coordinated, comprehensive national strategy."[43]

The center of that strategy is the reform of TSCA (toss-ka), the 1976 federal Toxic Substances Control Act, which has been a prime target of health and environmental advocates since the day it was implemented.

TSCA's fatal flaw, say public health experts, is that the burden of proving that a particular substance is toxic falls on the government, not on the industry that synthesized it. The US EPA, which is charged with regulating dangerous chemicals, gets only 90 days' notice to raise safety concerns about new chemicals or compounds before they can be introduced to the market, and manufacturers are not required to submit safety data if none exist.[44] In about 85 percent of new chemical notices, no safety data are submitted.[45]

Additionally, at the time the law was passed, about 60,000 chemicals were already in production, and no safety data were required for their continued approval.[46] These included a number of chemicals, including BPA and some polybrominated diphenyl ethers (PBDEs), a family of chemicals widely used as flame retardants in furniture and other products. PBDEs, which are structurally similar to PCBs and dioxin, have been banned in 150 signatory countries by the United Nation's Stockholm Convention on Persistent Organic Pollutants (which the United States has not signed) and by more than a dozen US states due to evidence that they may interfere with normal brain development in infants.[47]

In fact, in the nearly four decades since enactment of TSCA, the US EPA has required testing of only about 200 of the more than 82,000 chemicals on the market, and it has succeeded in restricting or limiting the use of a grand total of only five chemicals: PCBs (which were mandated in the original legislation), chlorofluorocarbons (CFCs), dioxins, hexavalent chromium, and asbestos, a proven carcinogen that, despite EPA use restrictions, remains a hazard for hundreds of thousands of workers in the construction and building maintenance industries.[48] The reason for the lack of testing? Before the agency can test a chemical for risk, it has to show that the product poses "unreasonable risk." In other words, the US EPA is bound in a classic Catch-22.

TSCA has been so ineffectual in protecting human and environmental health (see Box 6.2) that in 2009 the US Government Accountability Office (GAO) listed TSCA among the "high-risk" areas of government requiring immediate reform. According to the GAO report, "The EPA does not have sufficient chemical assessment information to determine whether it should establish controls to limit public exposure to many chemicals that may pose substantial health risks."[49]

Box 6.2   THE PRESIDENT'S CANCER PANEL

The President's Cancer Panel, in its May 2010 report on environmental cancer risks, refers to the TSCA as "the most egregious example of ineffective regulation of chemical contaminants."[50] Both the GAO and the Cancer Panel called for legislation that would put the burden of proof for the safety of new and existing chemicals on the chemical manufacturers rather than the regulators, the model that is standard for chemical regulation in the European Union.

Pressure to reform TSCA along the lines suggested by the green chemistry movement has drawn active support from throughout the environmental movement and the health care industry and related sectors. Representing Kaiser Permanente, I testified before Congress on two separate occasions regarding concerns we have with the existing law.[51] Dignity Health has put forward their own guidelines for TSCA reform, including the following:

- A minimum set of data, available to the public, on the health and environmental hazards for all chemicals in commerce within 5 years.
- Full safety determinations for all new chemicals before they are allowed to come to market, thus avoiding the industry's replacement of known toxics with unknown but potentially toxic alternatives.
- Immediate phase-out of all persistent, bioaccumulative and toxic (PBT) chemicals except for critical uses.
- Expedited action by the US EPA to reduce exposures to other toxic chemicals that can cause serious health problems, such as DEHP, PBDEs, and BPA.
- Federal support for safer alternatives through research into green chemistry and incentives favoring safer chemicals and products over those with known health hazards.

Many of the reform advocates have come together in the Safer Chemicals Healthy Families coalition to press for passage of federal reform legislation, which has stalled in Congress since it was first introduced in 2005. Reintroduced every year since by Sen. Lautenberg, who passed away after introducing a compromise version of the legislation in 2013, the Safe Chemicals Act would shift the burden back to the chemical industry to prove its products are safe, establish health standards for chemicals to protect children and other vulnerable groups, and strengthen the public's right to know about the safety and use of chemicals.

Nonetheless, TSCA reform advocates remain optimistic. They believe the tide has turned in favor of passage of a greener, safer federal chemicals policy, led by numerous states that have passed chemical safety laws by large, bipartisan margins in recent years. Equally important, a growing number of national retailers and consumer product manufacturers, including Whole Foods, Staples, Steelcase, Seventh Generation, Hewlett-Packard, WalMart,

---

Box 6.3 REACH'S IMPACT

In preparing the REACH legislation, the European Commission performed a projected impact assessment that concluded that full implementation of the law over 11 years would result in a 10 percent reduction of diseases caused by chemicals. If accurate, REACH would be responsible for avoiding roughly 4,500 deaths in the European Union (EU) due to cancer alone annually. In financial terms, the law's potential health benefit was estimated to total roughly 50 billion Euros (about $75 billion in 2008) over a 30-year period.[52]

A subsequent study in 2003, aimed at further strengthening REACH, reported that despite, or because of, the REACH regulations, Europe's chemical industry "has been strengthening its comparative advantage."[53] It also reported that between 1990 and 2000, the chemical industry's emissions of greenhouse gases from chemical processes fell by 50 percent, with production of ozone-depleting particles nearing zero. Acidifying gases (sulphur dioxide, ammonia, and nitrogen oxides) dropped by 48 percent, despite a 33 percent increase in chemical production.

and others are responding to consumer demands for safer, healthier prod-ucts by implementing their own safer-chemicals purchasing policies.

And finally, new international pressure is coming from the European Union, which implemented the most ambitious chemicals legisla-tion in the world in 2007, known as REACH (Registration, Evaluation, Authorization and restrictions of Chemicals) (see Box 6.3).

Managed by the European Chemicals Agency in Helsinki, REACH requires the registration of some 30,000 chemical substances, with full hazard and risk management data to be supplied by manufacturers to ensure their safe use. REACH's focus on a list of substances of very high concern is expected to have significant impact on chemical production and use in the United States, since US companies produce or import hun-dreds of chemicals designated as dangerous by REACH. These companies will thereby be directly impacted by the EU regulations.[54]

With state governments, the US multinational business community, and international regulators taking the lead, discussions about policy reform continue. And we can acknowledge Sir Percival Pott and the besooted child chimney sweeps who cast the first light on the hidden health hazards of industrial age chemicals.

CASE STUDIES IN THE GREENING OF HEALTH CARE CHEMICALS

Green Cleaning at Ridgeview Medical Center

Among the major sites of potentially hazardous chemicals in most hospi-tals are the closets containing janitorial and cleaning supplies. Products used for general cleaning and for infection control (disinfectants) have long been used in great volumes throughout hospital settings. However, in recent years, a growing body of evidence has shown that many clean-ing and disinfecting agents may have a wide range of unintended health impacts, especially respiratory disorders such as asthma.[55] Cleaning chemicals may also contribute to the pollution of outdoor air and water supplies, among other environmental impacts. In response, many health care organizations have adopted various green cleaning practices, including selection of nontoxic or less toxic cleaners, alternate methods of cleaning, and even changes in building design and operation and selection of interior materials that minimize the harmful health effects of cleaning while maintaining or improving cleanliness and sanitation for patient and staff safety.[56]

Ridgeview Medical Center, an independent, regional health care network and 109-bed acute care hospital serving Minneapolis, uses green cleaning as a strategic method to reduce their impact on the environment and safeguard the health of their patients, employees, and visitors.[57] Ridgeview utilizes the Centers for Disease Control and Prevention guidelines for appropriate cleanliness levels throughout the facility, depending on the use of different areas. Areas that have high infection risks, such as operating rooms or intensive care units, are treated to more stringent cleaning requirements than office settings, which are not disinfected. "Never dust with dynamite," says Todd Wilkening, facilities director.

In the selection of green (or less toxic) products, Ridgeview looks for third-party certification by Green Seal. In some areas, vinegar and water or soap and water are used to reduce the use of toxic chemicals. Ridgeview also tries to select high-concentration cleaning products that have minimal or no aerosolization or fragrances in order to minimize waste and improve indoor air quality.

Other important tactics involve interior design approaches that facilitate or reduce the need for cleaning: These include a well-designed ventilation system, finish materials that are easy to clean and maintain, and floor mats at building entrances.

The facility typically monitors costs of supplies, cleaning staff hours per square foot, hospital-acquired infection rates, employee illness, and job satisfaction. According to environmental services manager Paul Whittaker, "Based on the overall cost data, the cost of green cleaning is at or slightly above the historic level, and green cleaning is not a financial burden for the facility."

Phasing Out Halogenated Flame Retardants at
Kaiser Permanente

Kaiser Permanente purchases large amounts of medical furniture, such as exam tables, chairs, and stools, and waiting room furniture. To comply with the California technical bulletin 117, which requires certain flame retardancy for upholstered furniture, our furniture supplier, Midmark, along with many other furniture manufacturers, utilized a group of chemicals known as halogenated flame retardants (HFRs).

HFRs are among the groups of chemicals of concern that the organization has been working to eliminate from the products it purchases, including electronic devices. These chemicals have been linked to a number of negative health outcomes, including damage and interruption to the endocrine, reproductive, and thyroid systems and their functions.

In purchasing medical furniture, Kaiser Permanente used its sustainability scorecard to uncover information about the potential environmental and health impacts of products, including their chemical composition. This process revealed that among those firms bidding for the contract, Midmark had the fewest number of products that contained HFRs (13 percent of their product line) and the company was open to discussing future HFR elimination. Subsequently, Midmark agreed to partner with Kaiser Permanente to convert the remaining 13 percent of products that still contain HFR compounds to non-HFR foam padding by April 2016. That involves finding alternate foam padding, testing it for durability and strength, and creating a conversion plan for specific furniture products.

In addition to phasing out HFRs, over the past few years Kaiser Permanente has required Midmark and all other suppliers of furniture to utilize fabrics that were approved through the organization's Sustainable Fabrics Alliance. The Alliance worked to minimize the presence of persistent, bioaccumulative toxins that are sometimes used as stain-resistant and protective coatings on fabrics, including HFRs.

NOTES

1. K. H. Strange, *Climbing Boys: A Study of Sweeps' Apprentices 1772–1875* (London: Allison & Busby, 1982).
2. M. F. Denissenko, A. Pao, M. Tang, and G. P. Pfeifer, "Preferential Formation of Benzo[a]pyrene Adducts at Lung Cancer Mutational Hotspots in P53," *Science* 274, no. 5286 (October 18, 1996): 430–432.
3. US EPA, "Toxic Substances Control Act Inventory: Basic Information," http://www.epa.gov/oppt/existingchemicals/pubs/tscainventory/basic.html.
4. National Center for Chronic Disease Prevention and Health Promotion, "The Power of Prevention: Chronic Disease... The Public Health Challenge of the 21st Century (2009), http://www.cdc.gov/chronicdisease/pdf/2009-Power-of-Prevention.pdf; see also P. Grandjean, D. Bellinger, A. Bergman, et al. "The Faroes Statement: Human Health Effects of Developmental Exposure to Chemicals in Our Environment," *Basic and Clinical Parmacology and Toxicology* 102, no 2 (2008): 73–75.
5. Laura Wright Treadway, "Pure Chemistry," *OnEarth* (summer 2011), http://www.onearth.org/article/pure-chemistry.
6. A. Prüss-Ustün et al., "Knowns and Unknowns on Burden of Disease Due to Chemicals: A Systematic Review," *Environmental Health* 10 (2011): 9.
7. P. Landrigan et al., "Environmental Pollutants and Disease in American Children: Estimates of Morbidity, Mortality, and Costs for Lead Poisoning, Asthma, Cancer, and Developmental Disabilities," *Environmental Health Perspectives* 110, no. 7 (2002): 721–772; L. Trasande et al., "Reducing the Staggering Costs of Environmental Disease in Children, Estimated at $76.6 Billion in 2008," *Health Affairs* 30, no. 5 (May 2011): 863–870.
8. Lara B. McKenzie et al., "Household Cleaning Product-Related Injuries Treated in US Emergency Departments in 1990–2006," *Pediatrics* 126, no. 3 (September 2010): 509–516.
9. Premier Safety Institute, "Choosing Safer Products Helps Improve the Health of Communities," http://www.bizngo.org/static/ee_images/uploads/resources/bizngo-factsheets-premier.pdf.
10. US CDC, "Environmental Chemicals," http://www.cdc.gov/biomonitoring/environmental_chemicals.html.
11. Physicians for Social Responsibility, "Toxic Chemicals Found in Doctors and Nurses," press release, October 8, 2009.
12. Philip J. Landrigan and Lynn R. Goldman, "Children's Vulnerability to Toxic Chemicals: A Challenge and Opportunity to Strengthen Health and Environmental Policy," *Health Affairs* 30, no. 5 (May 2011): 842–850.
13. Sara Goodman of Greenwire, "New CDC Survey Tracks Mercury Levels in Americans," *New York Times*, December 11, 2009
14. President's Cancer Panel, "Annual Report 2008–2009, Reducing Environmental Cancer Risk: What We Can Do Now" (Bethesda, MD: President's Cancer Panel, 2010), vi.
15. Advisory Committee on Childhood Lead Poisoning Prevention, "Low Level Lead Exposure Harms Children: A Renewed Call for Primary Prevention" (January 4, 2012),

3, http://www.cdc.gov/nceh/lead/acclpp/final_document_030712.pdf; E. Skammeritz et al., "Asbestos Exposure and Survival in Malignant Mesothelioma: A Description of 122 Consecutive Cases at an Occupational Clinic," *International Journal of Occupational and Environmental Medicine (IJOEM)* 2, no. 4 (October 2011), http://www.theijoem.com/ijoem/index.php/ijoem/article/view/107/210.

16. Agency for Toxic Substances and Disease Registry, "Cigarette Smoking, Asbestos Exposure, and Your Health" (June 2006), http://www.atsdr.cdc.gov/asbestos/site-kit/docs/CigarettesAsbestos2.pdf.

17. US EPA, "Cleaning up the Nation's Toxic Waste Sites: Markets and Technology Trends" (2004), http://www.clu-in.org/download/market/2004market.pdf.

18. Committee on Pesticides in the Diets of Infants and Children, National Research Council, "Executive Summary," in *Pesticides in the Diets of Infants and Children* (Washington, DC: National Academies Press, 1993).

19. Landrigan, "Environmental Pollutants and Disease in American Children," 842.

20. Committee on Pesticides in the Diets of Infants and Children, 7.

21. Landrigan, "Environmental Pollutants and Disease in American Children," 843.

22. Environmental Working Group, "Body Burden: The Pollution in Newborns," July 14, 2005, http://www.ewg.org/research/body-burden-pollution-newborns.

23. Landrigan and Goldman, "Children's Vulnerability to Toxic Chemicals," 843.

24. J. P. Myers, "The Weight of Evidence," *San Francisco Medicine* (April 2010): 19–21; Feliz Grun and Bruce Blumberg, "Minireview: The Case for Obesogens," *Molecular Endocrinology* 23, no. 8 (2009): 1127–1134.

25. CAC, "DES Update, Consumers," http://www.cdc.gov/des/consumers/about/index.html.

26. National Institute of Environmental Health Sciences, "Bisphenol A," http://www.niehs.nih.gov/health/topics/agents/sya-bpa/.

27. Frederick S. vom Saal et al., "Chapel Hill Bisphenol A Expert Panel Consensus Statement: Integration of Mechanisms, Effects in Animals and Potential to Impact Human Health at Current Levels of Exposure," *Reproductive Toxicology* 23, no. 2 (August–September 2007): 131–138.

28. Kaiser Permanente, "Parental Exposure to BPA During Pregnancy Associated with Decreased Birth Weight in Offspring" press release, May 13, 2011, http://xnet.kp.org/newscenter/pressreleases/nat/2011/051311bpa4birthweight.html

29. Brendan Borrell, "Toxicology: The Big Test for Bisphenol A," *Nature* 464 (April 21, 2010): 1122–1124.

30. Sabrina Taverise, "FDA Makes It Official: BPA Can't Be Used in Baby Bottles and Cups," *New York Times*, July 17, 2012.

31. Science and Environmental Health Network, http://www.sehn.org/precaution.html

32. First formulated by Thomas Lindhqvist in a 1990 report to the Swedish Ministry of the Environment.

33. http://democrats.energycommerce.house.gov/sites/default/files/documents/Testimony-Gerwig-CTCP-Revisiting-TSCA-2009-2-26.pdf

34. US EPA, "Basics of Green Chemistry," http://www2.epa.gov/green-chemistry/basics-green-chemistry#definition.

35. US EPA, "Green Chemistry," http://www.epa.gov/greenchemistry/.

36. P. T. Anastas and J. C. Warner, *Green Chemistry: Theory and Practice* (New York: Oxford University Press, 1998), 30.

37. Navigant Research, "Green Chemistry," http://www.navigantresearch.com/research/green-chemistry.

38. US EPA, "New England Green Chemistry 2011/2012 Strategic Report" (2012), http://www.epa.gov/region1/greenchemistry/pdfs/2011-2012ExecSummary.pdf.

39. Berkeley Center for Green Chemistry, http://bcgc.berkeley.edu/mission.

40. Michael P. Wilson, keynote presentation, American Industrial Hygiene Conference and Exhibition, Indianapolis, May 17, 2011.

41. Environmental Defense Fund, "A Primer on Proposition 65," http://www.edf.org/health/primer-proposition-65.

42. Beveridge & Diamond, "Client Alert: Green Chemistry at the State Level" (May 5, 2010), http://www.bdlaw.com/assets/attachments/05-05-10%20BD%20Client%20Alert%20-%20State%20Green%20Chemistry.pdf.

43. California EPA, "Cal/EPA Applauds UC Report on Green Chemistry," press release, January 17, 2008.

44. Sarah A. Vogel and Jody A. Roberts, "Why the Toxic Substances Control Act Needs an Overhaul, and How to Strengthen Oversight of Chemicals in the Interim," *Health Affairs* 30, no. 5 (May 2001): 998–905.

45. David Andrews, "New Chemicals: Sell First, Test for Safety Later?" May 31, 2013, http://www.ewg.org/enviroblog/2013/05/new-chemicals-sell-first-test-safety-later.

46. Sarah A. Vogel and Jody A. Roberts, "Why the Toxic Substances Control Act Needs an Overhaul, and How to Strengthen Oversight of Chemicals in the Interim," *Health Affairs* 30, no. 5 (May 2001): 998–905.

47. Katharine Mieszkowski, "High Levels of Banned Chemicals Found in Pregnant Californians," *The Bay Citizen*, August 10, 2011, https://www.baycitizen.org/news/environmental-health/banned-chemicals-found-high-levels-women/; T. McDonald, "A Perspective on the Potential Health Risks of PBDEs," *Chemosphere* 46, no. 5 (2002): 745–755; P. O. Darnerud et al, "Polybrominated Diphenyl Ethers: Occurrence, Dietary Exposure, and Toxicology," *Environmental Health Perspectives* 109, supp. 1 (March 2001): 49–68; P. O. Darnerud, "Toxic Effects of Brominated Flame Retardants in Man and Wildlife," *Environment International* 29, no. 6 (2003): 841–853, cited in National Resource Defense Council, "Healthy Milk, Healthy Baby: Chemical Pollution and Mother's Milk," http://www.nrdc.org/breast-milk/pbde.asp.

48. US GAO, "High-Risk Series: An Update," GAO-09-271 (2009), http://www.gao.gov/new.items/d09271.pdf.

49. US GAO, "Chemical Regulation: Options for Enhancing the Effectiveness of the Toxic Substances Control Act," GAO-09-428T (February 26, 2009), http://www.gao.gov/new.items/d09428t.pdf.

50. President's Cancer Panel.

51. http://democrats.energycommerce.house.gov/sites/default/files/documents/Testimony-Gerwig-CTCP-Revisiting-TSCA-2009-2-26.pdf and http://www.epw.senate.gov/public/index.cfm?FuseAction=Files.View&FileStore_id=4acbc06b-7 5d1-41f8-b06b-e606bd681cfb

52. Available at http://ec.europa.eu/enterprise/sectors/chemicals/reach/index_en.htm

53. Extended Impact Assessment, "Commission Staff Working Paper," European Commission (Brussels, October 29, 2003).

54. Environmental Defense Fund, "Across the Pond: Accessing REACH's First Big Impact on US Companies and Chemicals (September 2008, updated January 2009), http://www.edf.org/sites/default/files/8538_Across_Pond_Report.pdf.

55. Ahmed A. Arifl and George L. Delclos, "Association Between Cleaning-Related Chemicals and Work-Related Asthma and Asthma Symptoms Among Healthcare Professionals," *Journal of Occupational & Environmental Medicine* 69 (2012): 35–40.

56. Air Resources Board, "Indoor Air Chemistry: Cleaning Agents, Ozone and Toxic Air Contaminants," April 2006, http://www.arb.ca.gov/research/single-project. php?row_id=60560.

57. Xiabo Quan, Anjali Joseph, and Matthew Jelen, "Green Cleaning in Healthcare: Current Practices and Questions for Future Research" (Health Care Research Collaborative, September 2001), http://www.noharm.org/lib/downloads/ cleaners/Green_Cleaning_in_Healthcare.pdf.

7

Environmentally Preferable Purchasing

What We Buy Matters

Many years ago, before we had a full-fledged environmental sustainability program at Kaiser Permanente, I was working with a team focused on waste minimization. We were looking for both operational changes and upstream interventions that could cost-effectively reduce the mountain of materials that health care organizations typically send to landfills and incinerators every day. Maybe because my own workspace was beginning to look like a landfill itself, with growing stacks of printouts and interoffice documents spilling over every flat surface, I began thinking about paper and the failed promise of the paperless office. I was not so naïve as to believe we could actually get rid of paper, but what if we were just to make a good dent in the huge volume of paper we used and discarded every day. A little research and some back-of-the-envelope math revealed the stunning fact that a mere 10 percent reduction in paper use (and therefore purchasing) across the entire organization would result in an annual savings of $10 million, in addition to saving a small forest and reducing the volume of waste and all the handling and space it requires. Greatly excited (and a little naïve), I proposed that we launch a system wide "$10 million paper campaign" that would, among other things, encourage staff to print documents only when necessary and set copiers to the "double-sided" printing default.

For various reasons—among them, competing leadership priorities and lack of staff resources—the campaign never got off the ground in those early days. But for me, it provided a dramatic reminder of the fact that what we buy and how we buy it matters a great deal. Virtually everything that goes into an organization's waste stream came in through the purchasing and supply chain. So even small changes in our purchasing policies could have significant impacts not only on costs but also on a whole range of sustainability goals: waste minimization, safer chemicals, energy conservation and efficiency, and healthy foods. In effect, purchasing provides a decision point at which it is possible to move upstream in the supply chain to address a wide range of environmental impacts instead of having to manage those impacts after they have occurred. It is really a form of preventive resource medicine, and it is usually far less costly in terms of health impacts, dollars, labor, technical complexity, and negative publicity than having to correct the downstream environmental health hazards.

Kaiser Permanente purchases roughly $13 billion a year in medical and nonmedical products of all kinds, including pharmaceuticals, building materials, and IT equipment. The US health care industry as a whole spends in excess of $200 billion a year on supplies.[1] That is a lot of purchasing power. In fact, it is roughly equivalent to the annual spending power of the more than 70 million Americans born into the so-called millennial generation, or "Gen Y," during the last two decades of the twentieth century.[2] Think about that. What if that entire generation of Americans could somehow tie their consumer spending to demands that the products and services they purchase be not only cost competitive and of high quality but also be environmentally friendly and sustainable throughout their life cycle, from extraction of raw materials to manufacturing and distribution, to use, maintenance, and disposal.

Manufacturers might grumble, they might make excuses, they might beg for more time. But eventually, the most innovative, market-sensitive companies would find ways to gain market share by meeting the demands of this powerful minority. And eventually other companies would follow suit. And perhaps the rest of the population, the retiring baby boomers, the Gen-Xers, and whatever cohort follows the Gen-Yers, would start demanding the same attributes of cost, quality, and sustainability in their consumer purchases.

Such a fantasy is not really so far-fetched. Long before my $10 million paper idea fired my own interest in the power of purchasing, the Carter Administration ushered in what would come to be known as environmentally preferable purchasing (EPP), focusing originally on, yes, paper. The 1976 Resource Conservation and Recovery Act mandated that all paper purchased by the federal government contain at least 30 percent recycled content.[3] In 1993, the Clinton Administration expanded on the act by ordering all federal agencies to consider a variety of factors in purchasing or designing any products or services, including the "elimination of virgin material requirement; use of recovered materials; reuse of product; life-cycle cost; recyclability; use of environmentally preferable products; waste prevention...and ultimate disposal."[4] It defined "environmentally preferable" as meaning "products or services that have a lesser or reduced effect on human health and the environment when compared with competing products or services that serve the same purpose."

That order applied to more than 60 federal agencies, which acquired the vast majority of the federal government's $350 billion a year spending in total goods and services through contracts.[5] Since then, many state and local governments have implemented similar purchasing policies, prompting more and more companies to retool their product design and manufacturing processes in order to meet the demands of the world's largest group of consumers, federal and state agencies. Companies like Anheuser-Busch, Canon, IBM, Sony, Volvo, Daimler-Chrysler, Patagonia, and others soon joined the bandwagon to produce and market green products to meet the growing sustainability demands of both institutional and individual consumers.

FLEXING HEALTH CARE'S PURCHASING MUSCLE

The Growth of Environmentally Preferable Purchasing

The health care industry was not far behind. Purchasing departments at a handful of major health systems, including Kaiser Permanente, had been including language on specific environmental attributes, such as recyclability, in their requests for proposals (RFPs) to product suppliers on a selective basis since the mid- to late 1990s. But the first really large-scale achievement for EPP in health care began with the 1998 mercury elimination campaign by Hospitals for a Healthy Environment (H2E), the predecessor of Practice Greenhealth.

As part of that multiyear campaign, H2E worked closely with the nation's largest group purchasing organizations (GPOs), third-party entities that today aggregate, negotiate, and manage more than 70 percent of all product purchasing for more than 95 percent of all acute care hospitals.[6] H2E helped to inform the GPOs about the health impacts of mercury-containing products and the availability of alternative products with equal or superior clinical performance. Meanwhile, a small number of large health systems, including Dignity Health, adopted purchasing policies that required their GPOs and other suppliers to identify all products that contained mercury and PVC and to purchase alternatives whenever possible.

By 2005, three of the five largest GPOs implemented mercury-free purchasing policies for all contracts in which an acceptable alternative product was available, while others focused specifically on eliminating mercury thermometers and sphygmomanometers (blood pressure measuring devices) from all their contracts. The result was a dramatic shift in the entire mercury medical product line, with the GPOs reporting that total sales of mercury devices were steadily decreasing while sales of mercury-free products were increasing.[7] At the same time, as demands for environmentally preferable products grew, the GPOs working with H2E expanded their EPP focus to target products containing latex, glutaraldehyde, ethylene oxide, and toxic cleaning chemicals, plus reprocessing and waste management services, and energy and water efficiency equipment.

As the entire business of health care purchasing grew ever more sophisticated through health system partnerships with the GPOs, the benefits of EPP spilled over from the handful of health care organizations that had formal EPP programs to the great majority of organizations that did not but that benefited anyway because their GPOs made environmentally preferable products available at competitive costs. And as more health systems chose to purchase from the GPOs' EPP lists of product offerings, costs became even more competitive, in many cases undercutting the traditional non-EPP product lines. The result, from the early 2000s on, was significant growth and maturation of the EPP approach as hospitals and health systems all across the country found they could purchase both medical and nonmedical products that significantly reduced costs involved in waste disposal, liability, and occupational health; improved their overall environmental impacts; and contributed to a healthier environment for their patients, employees, and communities.

Additionally, the cost savings and the environmental benefits provided great grist to health systems for positive public communications. The multistate Dignity Health system, for instance, noted in its 2010 annual *Social Responsibility Report* that simply by purchasing more reprocessed medical products, which allows single-use products to be sterilized and safely used for more than one patient, it had saved $5.6 million at its clinics and hospitals in California, Arizona, and Nevada.[8]

Standardizing Questions to Suppliers

The growth of EPP in health care reached what may have been a critical tipping point in 2011, when five GPOs sat down with representatives from Practice Greenhealth's new Greening the Supply Chain Initiative at the annual CleanMed conference. All together, the participating GPOs manage $135 billion worth of contracts for medical products for more than 4,000 hospitals and thousands of other health care organizations.[9] For several years, they had been working with Practice Greenhealth to devise solutions to the difficulty of responding to the growing number of health systems that were submitting their own unique lists of questions and requirements regarding the environmental attributes of medical products, making it extremely difficult for the GPOs to meet everyone's needs. To better rationalize the process, the participating GPOs agreed to adopt a powerful, standardized list of environmental questions that would be submitted to all product and services suppliers bidding on the GPOs' negotiated contracts. The 13 standardized questions from Practice Greenhealth (see Box 7.1) applied to virtually all the medical products and equipment used in hospitals, medical offices, and other facilities and covered a broad range of environmental concerns, ranging from the presence of various chemicals of concern to carcinogens and reproductive toxicants, recycled content and recyclability, and product reusability.[10]

Gary Cohen, president of Health Care Without Harm, hailed the tool's adoption for "sending a clear signal to suppliers that hospitals are looking for safer chemicals and greener products" and predicted it would "shift the entire health sector marketplace toward more sustainable products."[11]

Kaiser Permanente took special satisfaction in the release of the tool, which is now available through Practice Greenhealth to any and all public or private health care purchasers. In fact, the standardized questions were based almost word for word on our own first-in-the-nation Sustainability Scorecard, which we had begun using with our GPO, MedAssets, and other suppliers in 2010 to assess and track the environmental sustainability of our own $1 billion-plus annual spend on medical products. We already knew the Scorecard could move the market toward sustainability, and the more health systems that used it the faster we would all get there.

As Robert Gotto, then Kaiser Permanente's executive director of EPP and National Facility Services Procurement, observed, the $135 billion annual spending now going through the EPP standardized questions to GPOs and suppliers represents about 80 percent of all the medical products bought in this country. "That's a big chunk of the global business in medical products," says Gotto, "and this is why we shared our Sustainability Scorecard. When we have a win, we want everyone else to share in it, because what we really want is for the supply chain to move."[12]

Box 7.1 **PRACTICE GREENHEALTH'S STANDARDIZED ENVIRONMENTAL QUESTIONS FOR MEDICAL PRODUCTS, VERSION 1.0**

Medical products, for the purposes of this questionnaire, are defined as selected products used to diagnose, treat, or care for patients. Excluded are electronic medical products (anything that plugs in or has a battery) and pharmaceuticals.

1. Does this product contain postconsumer recycled content (excluding steel)? If yes, what percentage by weight?
2. Is this product recyclable?
3. Does the product's primary packaging contain postconsumer recycled content? If yes, what percentage?
4. Is this product packaged without polystyrene?
5. Is this product sold as a multiuse product or device (not single use)?
6. Is this product free of intentionally added polyvinyl chloride (PVC)?
7. Is this product free of intentionally added phthalates: DEHP, BBP, DnHP, DIDP, and DBP? If no, please specify the phthalate(s).
8. Is this product free of intentionally added Bisphenol A (BPA) or BPA-derived plastics (such as polycarbonate plastic and resins)?
9. Does this product contain less than 1000 ppm halogenated organic flame retardants by weight of homogenous material?
10. Is this product free of intentionally added mercury?
11. Is this product free of intentionally added latex?
12. Will this product be classified (on its own or when aggregated) as nonhazardous waste according to the Environmental Protection Agency's (EPA) RCRA (Resource Conservation and Recovery Act) when disposed? (under 40 CFR 261.31-33)?
13. Does this product contain carcinogens or reproductive toxicants, as listed under the California Safe Drinking Water and Toxic Enforcement Act of 1986, Proposition 65, below Proposition 65 Safe harbor levels?

That movement got another big boost in 2012 when the newly formed Healthier Hospitals Initiative (HHI) included environmentally preferable purchasing among the six major challenges the organization is urging on all the nation's hospitals. HHI itself is made up of many of the largest, most influential US health systems, comprising some 500 hospitals with more than $20 billion in purchasing power. The EPP challenge urges organizations to, at the very least, adopt Practice Greenhealth's standardized environmental questions for medical products in their GPO partnerships. It also urges them to commit to a variety of EPP actions, such as buying only electronic products certified by the Electronic Products Environmental Assessment Tool (EPEAT) and purchasing reprocessed single-use devices as a way to reduce waste.

With all this activity to propel the EPP strategy, it is tempting to believe that, one day soon, the procurement function of large health systems could single-handedly transform hospital environments into the safe, healthy, and environmentally friendly places that everyone wants and expects. But the fact is that EPP procurement is still very much a work in progress in the United States, lagging the participation levels reached by health systems in many European countries, where EPP policies tend to be developed on a national or even European Union–wide basis. EPP is regarded by many in health care's C-suite and purchasing departments as an interesting but lower priority add-on to other goals, chiefly financial. A 2012 survey of health care executives, including purchasing professionals, found that only about one in five respondents even knew whether their institution had an EPP program, although more than 90 percent of those who did have a program felt it was important in driving their purchasing decisions. Nonetheless, only about a quarter of US health systems responding to the survey reported that they had moved a product contract from one supplier to another on the basis of environmentally preferable attributes.[13] That leaves a lot of room for progress.

Additionally, as powerful as a well-designed EPP program can be, even the procurement professionals who embrace the strategy and tout its achievements are among the first to acknowledge that EPP may produce disappointing and even costly results unless it is well integrated into a multiprong, holistic sustainability strategy that spans an organization's entire operations.

As our own procurement leaders repeatedly remind us, simply purchasing environmentally preferable products and services does not guarantee that they will have an impact. For their potential to be realized, it is as much a question of how the products are used and maintained and treated at the end of their useful life by the doctors, nurses, lab techs, clerical workers, logistics personnel, food service workers, engineers, drivers, janitors, and scores of other workers who play essential roles in any successful sustainability strategy.

By the way, my campaign to save $10 million in paper purchases was not realized as originally proposed, but we have made significant progress. When our Procurement and Supply department published an internal article about our environmentally preferable purchasing (EPP) program in early 2008, they received a flood of positive responses from employees, many of whom provided valuable suggestions for improvement. The number-one suggestion was to commit to buying recycled-content (RC) copy paper and to completely eliminate the purchase of copy paper made only of virgin pulp (pulp straight from the forest). Thanks to the employee enthusiasm, we made the commitment and today we buy 2 million reams a year of 30 percent RC copy paper, which has presented no problems with our copiers and printers. The conversion was cost neutral, and the life-cycle savings of the RC paper has saved more than 10 million gallons of water, 36,000 trees per year (equivalent to all the trees in New York's Central Park), and 6.2 million kilowatt-hours of electricity, enough to serve 5,500 average US homes. We also worked with our printer equipment supplier and our IT people to standardize printer settings to reduce paper consumption and engaged employees to reduce printing.

The Kaiser Permanente Environmentally Preferable Purchasing Model: How It Works

Kaiser Permanente is certainly not the only large health system in the United States that has been practicing increasingly sophisticated environmentally preferable purchasing for close to two decades. But it is reasonably safe to assert that most health systems looking to undertake or expand their own EPP programs look to the experience of Kaiser Permanente and a few other longtime EPP champions as models to learn from.

That said, some of what Kaiser Permanente does may not be practical for other health systems. Kaiser Permanente does have one capability that has been the major enabler of their EPP successes; they are a fully integrated health care system, in which physicians, hospitals, and the health plan have successfully come together to pursue a common mission to optimize financial and quality goals. In other words, the EPP program benefits from the power of system wide collaboration and cooperation. This capability is not developed among less integrated systems, in which physicians, hospital administrators, and insurance executives are often at odds over medical product purchasing. On the other hand, it probably is also true that smaller systems are able to act on purchasing opportunities with greater speed and flexibility than a system of 38 hospitals and 9.1 million members scattered across seven geographic regions. Being big can have its drawbacks.

Kaiser Permanente has been practicing some level of EPP since at least the mid-1990s, when we were among the first systems to embrace Health Care Without Harm's campaigns against mercury and PVC (discussed in Chapter 1), which we approached as both a procurement issue and an internal operations challenge. In those days, all our purchasing was done internally. But in 2001 we began partnering with a large GPO called Broadlane (since merged into MedAssets) to negotiate more favorable national contracts for medical, surgical, business, and some IT products. By joining with Broadlane's other health system partners, we were able to leverage our combined purchasing strength to save a total of $55 million on national contracts annually by 2003, and to lower our procurement overhead by some $5 million annually by outsourcing to the GPO many of the functions of our National Purchasing Organization. Other health systems have realized comparable savings for their size.

What we did not outsource was the decision-making function over the more than $1 billion in medical products that we purchase through the GPO. That critical function remained with our National Product Council, a group of senior physicians, nurses, and health plan executives that oversees

35 specialty-focused sourcing and standards teams (SSTs). These teams are composed of clinicians with special expertise in their fields, which include orthopedics, cardiology, medical imaging, physiological monitoring, sharps safety, medical endoscopy, urology, and so on. They are responsible for conducting product trials and gathering other evidence on the clinical quality, regulatory compliance, assurance of supply, supplier service, innovation, and total lifetime cost of all medical products in their areas of specialization. Working with consultants from the GPO and from our own Procurement and Supply organization, the SSTs make evidence-based recommendations on product standardization to the National Product Council. Similar product evaluation teams perform parallel functions for some $6 billion in annual spending on nonmedical products, including everything from automobiles to zucchini. Pharmaceutical purchasing, which amounts to another roughly $6 billion annually, is managed through a similar but separate evidence-based approach.

The SSTs, says Robert Gotto, are able to make incredibly bold decisions because they have all the different clinical and nonclinical functions represented, they collect extensive data that enables them to uncover and evaluate new options, and the team stays together though implementation—learning from their failures and gaining confidence from their successes, thereby minimizing the extent of nonstandard and non-evidence-based "physician preference" purchases—a problem that bedevils many health care organizations. "These teams," he continues, "time and again are driving 20 to 30 percent cost reductions because they're able to look at the supplier and say, 'We've evaluated your product's clinical performance and our data shows that the cost premium you are proposing is significantly out of line with the market.'"

Environmental sustainability considerations in product purchasing were limited in the early years of this arrangement to certain high-priority product categories such as all products used in the neonatal intensive care units. The procurement department personnel assisting the SSTs were responsible for informing the clinical teams about the environmental attributes of products, and the clinicians would factor that information into their overall assessments when recommending a product for purchase. Although factors like clinical quality and supplier service are important, the environmental "score" of a product can often surprisingly prove to be the decisive factor in awarding a contract. That is because the majority of medical products (such as surgical instruments, pacemakers, monitors, beds) have been available for several years and are well along in their product maturity cycle, which means that there is now minimal product differentiation among the major manufacturers, and their products are often roughly comparable in terms of price, quality, and service. "When all the products are basically the same, that's an opportunity for some supplier to get ahead of their competitors and innovate by addressing these 'new' environmental factors, such as toxicity or recyclability," says Gotto. "And when that happens, then the sustainability performance actually becomes the only differentiator and therefore the decision point to award business to that supplier."

The scope of EPP in procurement quickly expanded and grew in importance with the creation of our Environmental Stewardship Council, a formal leadership group for sustainability activities across the entire system, thanks to the fact that the purchasing department was one of the council's chief sponsors. Also, our purchasing leaders strongly endorsed the council's adoption of the Precautionary Principle as a key sustainability guideline: "Where there is credible evidence that a material we're using may result in environmental or public health harm, we should strive to replace it with safer alternatives." This, in effect, provided the foundation for an increasingly ambitious and focused EPP program over the next few years, even though, like many other health systems that have embraced EPP, we did not at the time (late 1990s) have a formal system wide EPP policy or dedicated leadership.

By the time we developed a written policy on EPP in 2006, we already had established clear sustainability priority areas for product purchasing, spelled out in separate, formal policies on the use of chemicals; healthy, sustainably produced food; and other environmental priorities. What the EPP policy did for us, among other things, was provide a vehicle for communicating our EPP goals both internally, among users of the products, and externally to the GPO and suppliers. And because it would be impractical to focus the policy on specific products—we purchase some 200,000 distinct products and services—the policy addresses the environmental issues that we wanted to target for all the products we purchase. These issues included our four priority categories: chemicals of concern: healthy, sustainably produced food; energy and natural resources consumption; and waste minimization—all areas we had been working on for more than a decade.

The Sustainability Scorecard

The next big step in the evolution of the process was to find a relatively simple way to inform suppliers about our environmental expectations for products, not at the product category level but on a product-by-product basis. We had to go from asking, "Is there mercury in *these* products?" to asking, "Is there mercury in *this* product?"

The solution, developed over several years and with plenty of input from the major suppliers, was the Sustainability Scorecard, initially launched in October 2009, with an expanded second-generation version launched 18 months later. The Scorecard does not cover every environmental attribute we might like to know about, but it does cover the key data points that we knew the suppliers could provide, not only about medical products but also about the environmental practices of the supplier organizations themselves.

The scorecard enables us to gather the facts about individual products and hand that off to the SSTs so that they can make informed choices based on data. A few years ago, we had very little idea what the environmental impacts were between one product and another, but this gives us the facts right up front so we can make the best decision. It is an incredibly powerful tool.

Embedding Environmentally Preferable Purchasing into the Organizational DNA

It may seem impractical for a health care provider to spend valuable time and resources collecting and managing data on the chemical composition, recyclability, and life-cycle ecological impacts (not to mention the corporate social responsibility profile of product manufacturers and distributors) of 200,000 or more products and services. And that is in addition to collecting and analyzing all the other data we were already demanding on product quality, total cost of ownership, supplier service, and assurance of supply. However, that is exactly what our policy committed us to do, and we have managed it with surprisingly few additional resources. The main costs have been limited to the addition of a position to manage the EPP process in the areas of medical supplies, nonmedical supplies, IT, and food, plus some additional training in EPP for the procurement and supply teams. For the training, we partnered with EPP experts at Practice Greenhealth.

It is all possible because we were able to offload much of the burden of data collection and processing to our GPO, which has the data-crunching capability to manage the incoming tide of product information we request in our RFPs. Also, those 200,000 separate products that Kaiser Permanente purchases are not procured through individual contracts, but through as few as 1,000 separate contracts, each of which may cover 100 or more products in a category, and each of which extends for 3–5 years.

Rachael Baker, who managed Kaiser Permanente's EPP program for several years, notes that another factor enabling a smooth transition into a successful program was that "an ethic of sustainability was already part of the DNA of the entire organization," thanks to a mission that emphasized health in its broadest sense. That mindset, she adds, became even more embedded among the procurement and supply teams when a focus on environmental purchasing became part of the formal annual performance review process for procurement employees—something that may be unique to Kaiser Permanente, according to external EPP champions. "We're all responsible for delivering environmental excellence within the purview of our jobs," says Baker. "So whether you're a transportation person or someone purchasing a billion dollars' worth of stuff, it's your responsibility to find a way to promote sustainability, and most of us think that's a really cool thing. It expands the vision of our work."

To support broader learning from our own experiences, the procurement department put together over 40 one-page case studies of EPP outcomes and shared them through Kaiser Permanente's communications and on Practice Greenhealth's website. We share this information broadly as a contribution to improving the health of the communities we serve.

Pointing the Way to Greener Capitalism

How does cost figure into the process? Cost, like quality, is always a prime consideration in purchasing decisions, but not just the upfront purchase price.

"We have to look at things from the total cost of ownership perspective," says Vanessa Lochner, our director of EPP. From that perspective, reductions in waste or reducing consumption of natural resources, such as water, will almost always produce cost benefits (see Box 7.2). The same is true for reducing energy consumption. Reductions in use of toxic chemicals and heavy metals will not always produce cost savings, but nearly all of the product conversions we have made to reduce harmful chemicals have produced a cost reduction as well.

Box 7.2 SAVINGS THROUGH ENVIRONMENTALLY PREFERABLE PURCHASING

According to a carefully vetted analysis of Kaiser Permanente's procurement and supply operations from 2009 through 2011, the EPP program delivered $63 million in annualized savings while reducing energy consumption by 87 million kilowatt hours, reducing/recycling/reusing 12,000 tons of waste, reducing water use by 118 million gallons, reducing fuel use by 457,000 gallons, and substantially reducing consumption of hazardous metals and toxic chemicals.

"The vast majority of times, we're able to drive an environmental benefit and get a cost savings on top of it," says Lochner. "But it's absolutely critical to factor in the total cost of ownership," including the cost or savings involved in maintenance, cleanup of hazardous spills, reusability, recyclability, or disposal.

Indeed, major environmental benefits and cost savings are happening across the health care landscape as more and more health systems, both small and large, adopt the supplier questionnaire through Practice Greenhealth and engage in the Healthier Hospitals Initiative's purchasing challenge. In 2012, the 149 hospitals and health systems that received awards for outstanding sustainability practices at Practice Greenhealth's CleanMed conference boasted a combined annual savings of $55 million through product recycling, energy and water conservation, and avoided waste generation.[14] Not all, but much of that was thanks to environmentally preferable purchasing decisions.

As Baker put it, "This is how capitalism works. We (the hospitals) tell the suppliers where we want to go, and they will eventually get there. But we have to model the way."

TARGETING ENVIRONMENTALLY PREFERABLE PURCHASING FOR ITS GREATEST IMPACTS

So far, this chapter has focused on EPP's potential to accelerate the transformation of the health care products marketplace toward environmental sustainability and how the strategy has evolved and been shared by Kaiser Permanente. Now I want to turn to the work itself—where the strategy is already proving itself and where further opportunities exist in hospitals and health systems for driving the sustainability agenda through purchasing practices while reaping cost savings.

Ultimately, we need to look at virtually every product we buy, use, and eventually discard. But some products are more wasteful than others, some more hazardous than others, some have greater impacts on the environment than others, and some have more direct impacts on individual and community health than others. So it is useful in implementing an EPP program to perform strategic risk and opportunity assessments to identify the most problematic products or product categories, along with those that provide the biggest total return in each of the priority areas of the overall sustainability strategy.

These priority areas may differ in number and scope from one organization to another depending on the type of operations and geographic locations. As I have said, at Kaiser Permanente our priorities are safer chemicals and materials, waste minimization, sustainable energy, water conservation, and sustainable food. On the basis of strategic assessments by the procurement staff and the Environmental Stewardship Council, we set annual and long-term targets in each of these areas.

For food, we are striving to increase the purchase of sustainable food choices to at least 20 percent of our total food purchases by the end of 2015 from the 15 percent level we achieved in 2011, focusing especially on increasing sustainable options for protein foods, such as cage-free egg products.

In the chemicals area, our goal is to contract for safer alternatives to high-priority products. From 2009 to 2013 we targeted 10 products and contracted for safer alternatives to IV tubing and solution bags, dialysis bags and tubing, high-level disinfectants, enzymatic detergents, janitorial cleaning chemicals, cabinetry and casework, paint, resilient flooring, infant soaps and lotions, and adult and infant mattresses.

In the energy and natural resources area, our goal is to reduce our absolute greenhouse gas emissions by 30 percent by 2020, compared to the 2008 baseline. That requires increasing the energy efficiency of our new and existing facilities as well as purchasing both onsite and off-site renewable electricity generation, which we are pursuing by steadily increasing our capacity in solar and wind power. As a major consumer of municipal water, we also focused on water conservation efforts, including implementation of rainwater harvesting at some facilities, dual-flush toilets, gray water reuse, and drought-resistant landscaping. We have already made gains in water use thanks to our switch to digital diagnostic imaging equipment, which enhances image analysis and does not require the large amounts of water and chemicals needed for traditional X-ray film processing.

Health care organizations with less experience in EPP purchasing might well choose less ambitious goals as they learn to ramp up their programs. An excellent starting point would be any or all of the three EPP priority areas promoted by the Healthier Hospitals Initiative. These include two major waste reduction strategies—reformulation of surgical kits and reprocessing of single-use medical devices, which is covered in Chapter 5—and implementation of the Electronic Products Environmental Assessment Tool (EPEAT). The EPEAT strategy goes after waste as well, including disposal of toxic chemicals, but it also includes positive impacts on consumption of energy, natural materials, and greenhouse gas emissions.

Minimizing E-Waste Through Smart Purchasing

Computers and related IT devices are revolutionizing health care, improving quality, preventing medical errors, increasing administrative efficiencies, and—contrary to early fears—increasing patient-centeredness. Kaiser Permanente's recently retired Chairman and CEO, George Halvorson, one of the nation's leading advocates of electronic medical records and other e-connectivity tools, has called the computer "possibly the single most important tool available to health care."[15]

But computers and assorted other electronic devices, whether in health care or banking, manufacturing or home use, also have a dark side. Given the phenomenal growth rate of IT devices and their shrinking life spans, they now constitute the fastest growing portion of the nation's waste stream, at almost three times the growth rate of municipal waste.[16] And due to poor, largely unregulated waste management practices and a largely ineffective patchwork of state-level regulations on e-waste disposal and recycling—and no federal regulations—their disposal in landfills or incinerators is poisoning the air and ground water. It is threatening human health all over the world with a witch's brew of known or suspected reproductive toxins, endocrine disrupters, mutagens, persistent bioaccumulative substances, and carcinogens. In short, they have become one of the most environmentally challenging product categories of our time.

Health care organizations, as an increasingly large-volume purchaser of computers and electronic devices, have a special responsibility to use its purchasing power to move the electronics market toward safer, greener practices throughout the entire lifecycle of these products, from manufacture to use to end-of-life disposal. The major environmental and health challenges of electronic products fall into three principal categories.

TOXIC SUBSTANCES

Health care organizations purchase many billions of dollars' worth of computers, electrocardiogram monitors, and other electronic bio-medical devices every year, and much of this life-saving equipment, especially older models, contains hazardous substances. The average computer, for instance, is made up of more than 1,000 individual components, the raw materials of which represent most of the elements of the periodic table. PVCs show up in cable wiring, cadmium in batteries and resistors, lead in cathode ray tubes, mercury in LCD lights, and brominated flame retardants in plastic computer circuit boards and computer housing.[17]

Although users of these products are rarely, if ever, exposed to the toxic components of these products, other individuals at both ends of the products' lifecycle—extraction industries and manufacturing companies, as well as recycling and waste disposal workers—are at risk. And the health impacts can be severe, including birth defects, neurological problems, cancer, and hormonal imbalances.[18]

WASTE GENERATION

The greatest danger of contamination, however, comes from inappropriate disposal at the end of the products' ever-shorter life spans. The US EPA estimates that in 2009 US consumers and businesses discarded 2.4 million tons of computers, TVs, cell phones, and hard copy peripherals (including printers, scanners, and fax machines), and only a little more than a quarter of that waste was collected for recycling, with the remainder disposed of in landfills.[19] A study of solid waste in California indicated that some 70 percent of all the heavy metals, including lead, mercury, and cadmium, in landfills came from electronic products.[20] That was before California became of one the first states to pass an e-waste recycling law in 2003. Since then, about 25 other states have passed e-waste recycling regulations, but they differ widely in the scope of products covered, and most of them do not forbid brokers from shipping devices overseas. When improperly disposed, these products can release their hazardous substances to contaminate ground water and pollute the air, and the liability attaches directly to the end user, not the product manufacturer.

Even more serious threats to environmental and human health may come from the 50 to 80 percent of US e-waste that is collected for recycling and dismantled in US prisons or exported, mostly to informal recycling networks in developing countries,[21] where untrained workers who disassemble the products to salvage valuable components are often not protected from contamination.

Energy Use

It is hard to find reliable information on the current energy footprint of computers and related devices, but there is no question it is oversized and growing. Back in 1999 when the World Wide Web was still in its infancy, researchers at the Lawrence Berkeley National Laboratory examined energy consumption by what was already an exploding market in electronic office equipment and network equipment. They estimated total direct energy use by these devices was roughly 2 percent of total US electricity use. When they added in power use by telecommunications equipment and electronics manufacturing, the total shot up to 3 percent of all electricity use.[22] In a much narrower study, focusing just on the energy consumption of US computer data servers and the facilities that house them—not including the computers they actually serve—the National Resource Defense Council estimated that they consume more than 75 billion kWh annually, equivalent to the output of 26 medium-sized coal-fired power plants—and that half of that energy is wasted.[23]

Purchasing Strategies for Greener Electronics

Growing awareness of the environmental and health hazards posed by the growing use of computers and other electronic devices in health care has spurred development of a variety of tools and strategies to drive the market toward a greener future, and many of these are being incorporated into purchasing contracts. Nonprofit organizations like the Computer Takeback Campaign, Practice Greenhealth, and the Green Electronics Council all feature extensive advice and toolkits for healthier electronics purchasing on their websites.

The Electronic Product Environmental Assessment
Tool and Beyond

The most significant development of the past decade has been the creation in 2006 of the Electronic Product Environmental Assessment Tool (EPEAT), mentioned earlier. EPEAT is an EPA-funded set of voluntary but stringent environmental criteria for more than a thousand electronic products. It provides a system for helping institutional buyers, such as hospitals, avoid the deceptive marketing practices, known as "greenwashing," by some product manufacturers by identifying and verifying products that meet its criteria (see Box 7.3).

EPEAT's environmental rating system evaluates computers, laptops, monitors, and other equipment on 51 environmental issues, and it awards three levels of certification to manufacturers—bronze, silver, and gold—for products that satisfy most or all of the criteria. The 51 EPEAT standards, 23 of which are required for the lowest certification level, cover eight categories:

- Reduction or elimination of environmentally sensitive materials, including compliance with the European Union's Restriction of the use of certain Hazardous Substances (RoHS), including heavy metals

Box 7.3 HOW TO AVOID "GREENWASHING"

As environmentally preferable purchasing catches on among US health care organizations, some product manufacturers and retailers are bending over backward to promote their eco-friendliness. These vendors spend more on eco-marketing, or "greenwashing" (making deceptive promotional claims about a product's environmental characteristics), than on ensuring that their products are as environmentally preferable as they claim to be.

How can a conscientious purchaser stay ahead of the marketing rhetoric without having to be an expert in all things green? The US Environmental Protection Agency offers a number of tools to facilitate reliable environmentally preferable purchasing at www.epa.gov/epp. Practice Greenhealth's website at www.practicegreeenhealth.com offers lots of helpful advice, including a list of reliable third-party product certifications covering hundreds of product categories and various environmental attributes. Some of the most common and reliable certifications to look for include the following:

- **EPAT:** Electronic Products Environmental Assessment Tool. This is an independent program that certifies green electronic equipment such as computers, monitors, and laptops. http://www.epeat.net.
- **Energy Star:** A joint program of the US Department of Energy and the US Environmental Protection Agency (EPA) that lists qualified energy-efficient products (such as lighting, exit signs, appliances, and office equipment). http://www.energystar.gov.
- *e*-**Stewards:** A nonprofit organization that certifies electronic recyclers who recycle in an environmentally responsible manner, including not sending electronics to developing countries, not landfilling or incinerating materials, and not using prison labor to recycle electronic parts. http://www.e-stewards.org.
- **Green Seal:** A nonprofit organization that set standards through a multistakeholder, consensus-based process for products (such

as janitorial cleaners, floor strippers, and paints) and services (including hotels and cleaning services) and certifies they meet those standards. http://www.greenseal.org.

- **Green-e:** A labeling program established by the nonprofit organization Center for Resource Solutions, which verifies through its Green-e Energy label that electricity that has been generated using renewable sources such as solar and wind energy. http://www.green-e.org.

- **Greenguard:** A nonprofit organization that certifies products with reduced impact on indoor air quality (those with low volatile organic compounds or VOCs). Certified products include flooring, paints, commercial furniture, and cleaning products. Some labels reflect varying levels of impact on air quality. Prefer GREENGUARD "Children and Schools" and the new "Premier" label for the lowest indoor air impacts. http://www.greenguard.org.

- **Scientific Certification Systems:** A private company that certifies a variety of green claims, including "Recycled content," "Organic," or low volatile organic compounds (VOCs). http://www.scscertified.coms.

- **US Department of Agriculture (USDA):** Developed national standards for organically produced agricultural products to assure consumers that agricultural products marketed as organic meet consistent, uniform standards on the use of pesticides and fertilizers and other approved methods used to grow, harvest, and process food and other agricultural products. http://www.ams.usda.gov/AMSv1.0/.

- Materials selection, including percentage of recycled and biobased content
- Design for end-of-life disposition (recyclability)
- Life cycle extension (upgradability)
- Energy conservation, including compliance with the US EPA's Energy Star efficiency rating system

- End-of-life management, including product take-back provisions and auditing of recycling vendors
- Corporate performance, including written environmental policy and third-party certification for environmental management
- Packaging, including reusability, 90 percent recyclability, and a take-back provision; thanks to federal Executive Order 13423, 95 percent of all electronic products purchased by federal agencies must be EPEAT certified, and the same is true for many state and local governments.[24] Use of EPEAT standards has been growing at an impressive rate, up 30 percent in 2011 to more than 120 million units, including 25 percent of all PC sales worldwide.[25] The certification of those products over their lifetime, compared to non-EPEAT products, will reduce use of primary materials by an estimated 4.4 million metric tons, reduce use of toxic substances by nearly 1,400 metric tons, eliminate the volume of mercury equivalent to more than 1 million mercury thermometers, and avoid the disposal of more than 74,000 metric tons of hazardous waste. In addition, they will save more than 12 billion kWh of electricity— enough to power nearly a million US homes for a year—and reduce more than 2.2 metric tons of greenhouse gas emissions, equivalent to taking 1.6 million average US automobiles off the road for a year.[26]

Kaiser Permanente is firmly committed to the EPEAT standards, having been the first health care organization to adopt them back in 2006, when they were originally launched. We estimate that our EPEAT-registered computers saved us close to $5 million annually over the lifecycle of those products.[27] Today, over 95 percent of the desktops, monitors, and laptops we purchase meet the top EPEAT certification level. In 2013 EPEAT was also launched for printers and photocopiers, and Kaiser Permanente immediately adopted these standards as well, setting aggressive timelines with suppliers for EPEAT gold products.

EPEAT and additional IT purchasing practices got an even greater boost within the health care industry in 2010. Kaiser Permanente joined with Dignity Health, the big hospital group Premier, and our GPO, then known as Broadlane, to throw our combined weight behind an endorsement of the Center for Environmental Health's Guidelines for Environmentally Preferable IT Purchasing and Management. The announcement was timed to influence an expected boost in IT purchasing and disposal of legacy systems by hospitals and medical practices in the wake of the federal government's 2009 economic stimulus legislation, which provided nearly $20 billion in electronics purchasing subsidies to encourage health care organizations to adopt electronic health record systems.

The Center for Environmental Health's IT purchasing guidelines include the following:

- EPEAT registration, energy-efficiency labeling, halogen-free products, and products from producers with take-back programs
- Responsible use of electronics, including extending the life span and taking steps to minimize energy consumption
- Ensuring proper disposal of outdated equipment, including working with recyclers and waste management companies with E-Steward certification, which is awarded to firms that abide by the strongest international environmental and health regulations and standards
- Communicating a preference for safer electronics to suppliers[28]

The announcement of the guidelines came at the same time that Kaiser Permanente announced the sharing of its Sustainability Scorecard for medical products (discussed previously) and served as an important next step by extending EPP's scope to the IT sector. Adoption of the scorecard and the Center for Environmental Health (CEH) guidelines by Broadlane meant that the standards became available to all of its health care clients, including more than 1,100 acute care hospitals and 50,000 non–acute care facilities. The guidelines were also adopted by Premier, a hospital improvement alliance of more than 2,300 nonprofit hospitals and health systems, including Dignity Health, which had already adopted the EPEAT tool and the E-Steward commitment on e-waste management.

"A call for safer electronics and better e-waste management isn't just good for the environment and human health, it's also good for business," declared Sue Chiang, Pollution Prevention Program Director at CEH. "As electronic records become the industry standard, this marks a paradigm shift in the way the health care sector views their role around electronic purchasing, management, and disposal."[29]

The success of that paradigm shift toward safer, healthier electronics still depends in part on federal action to address the abuses of e-waste recyclers and to establish consistent, national regulations on the disposal of used electronics. So far, there is no federal mandate covering recycling of e-waste, although at least 25 states, covering roughly two thirds of the US population, have passed laws governing electronic product disposal since 2003.

NOTES

1. Practice Greenhealth, "Environmentally Preferable Purchasing," https://practice-greenhealth.org/topics/epp.
2. Judith Aquino, "Gen Y: The Next Generation of Spenders," *CRM*, February 1, 2012, http://www.destinationcrm.com/Articles/Editorial/Magazine-Features/Gen-Y-The-Next-Generation-of-Spenders-79884.aspx.
3. Jerrell D. Coggburn and Dianne Rahm, "Environmentally Preferable Purchasing: Who Is Doing What in the United States?" Journal of Public Procurement 5, no. 1 (2005): 23–53.
4. Executive Order no. 12873, "Acquisition, Recycling, and Waste Prevention" (October 20, 1993), http://www.epa.gov/epp/pubs/eo12873.pdf.
5. US EPA, "Environmentally Preferable Purchasing, Basic Information," http://www.epa.gov/epp/pubs/about/about.htm.
6. Healthcare Supply Chain Association, "A Primer on Group Purchasing Organizations," http://c.ymcdn.com/sites/www.supplychainassociation.org/resource/resmgr/research/gpo_primer.pdf.
7. Ibid.
8. Dignity Health, "Sustaining Our Healing Ministry: FY 2011 Social Responsibility Report 2010."
9. Johnson & Johnson, "The Growing Importance of More Sustainable Products in the Global Health Care Industry" (2012), 5, http://www.jnj.com/sites/default/files/pdf/JNJ-Sustainable-Products-White-Paper-092512.pdf.
10. Practice Greenhealth, "Standardized Questions for Environmental Purchasing," http://practicegreenhealth.org/gsc/standardized.

11. Health Care Without Harm, "New Tool to Assess Environmental Attributes of Medical Products," press release, October 13, 2011.

12. Robert Gotto, interviewed by the author, 2011.

13. Johnson & Johnson, "The Growing Importance."

14. Practice Greenhealth, "2012 Sustainability Benchmark Report," https://practice-greenhealth.org/tools-resources/sustainability-benchmark-report-0.

15. Lola Butcher, "George Halvorson Tells Me About the Perfect System," Health Care Payment Reform (blog), November 12, 2008, http://lolabutcher.com/wordpress/archives/27.

16. Health Care Without Harm and the Computer TakeBack Campaign, "Environmentally Preferable Procurement Guidelines for Information Technology Equipment in Health Care, Part I: The Issue," https://practicegreenhealth.org/pubs/Pub7-02-TheIssue.pdf.

17. Green Electronics Council, "The Connection Between Electronics and Sustainability," Green Electronics Council, http://greenelectronicscouncil.org/programs/research/.

18. US EPA, "Cleaning up Electronic Waste (E-Waste)," http://www.epa.gov/oiamount/toxics/ewaste/index-uew.html#ewastetabs.

19. Ibid.

20. Global Futures Foundation, "Computers, E-Waste, and Product Stewardship: Is California Ready for the Challenge?" Report for the US Environmental Protection Agency, Region IX, May 1, 2001, http://infohouse.p2ric.org/ref/41/40164.htm.

21. Greenpeace USA, "Where Does E-Waste Go?" http://www.greenpeace.org/usa/en/campaigns/toxics/hi-tech-highly-toxic/e-waste-goes/.

22. Kaoru Kawamoto et al, "Electricity Used by Office Equipment and Network Equipment in the US," Energy 27, no. 3 (March 2002), 255–269.

23. NRDC, "Are There Ghosts in Your Closet? Saving Wasted Energy in Computer Server Rooms" (2012), http://www.nrdc.org/energy/files/Saving-Energy-Server-Rooms-FS.pdf.

24. Executive Order 13423, "Strengthening Federal Environmental, Energy, and Transportation," Federal Register 72, no. 17 (January 26, 2007).

25. Healther Clancy, "Sales of EPEAT Registered Products Grew More Than 30 Percent in 2011," Green Tech Pastures, November 21, 2012, http://www.zdnet.com/sales-of-epeat-registered-products-grew-30-percent-in-2011-7000007742/.

26. Green Electronics Council, "Environmental Benefits of 2011 EPEAT Purchasing," Executive Summary (2011), 5.

27. "Kaiser Permanente Named Green Electronics Champion by EPA, Green Electronics Council," Kaiser Permanente press release, October 2, 2007.

28. Greener Computing Staff, "Healthcare Heavyweights Back IT Purchasing Standards," Greenbiz.com, May 13, 2010, http://www.greenbiz.com/news/2010/05/13/healthcare-heavyweights-back-it-purchasing-standards.

29. Center for Environmental Health, "Healthcare Giants Endorse Environmental Standards for Electronic Equipment," press release, May 10, 2010, http://www.ceh.org/news-events/press- releases/content/healthcare- giants-endorse- strong-environmental-standards-for- electronic-equipment/.

8

Greening the Built Health Care Environment

On a sunny day in the spring of 2013, I flew into Portland, Oregon, to tour Kaiser Permanente's newest hospital, the Westside Medical Center. It was still months before the 126-bed hospital was scheduled to open to patients, but it was late enough into the 36-month construction process that patient rooms were mostly furnished, walls were freshly painted, the campus grounds were neatly landscaped, and the central utility plant pumped heat through the buildings.

The hospital is Kaiser Permanente's first Leadership in Energy and Environmental Design (LEED®) Gold-certified hospital, and it earned big points for its open campus, which blends harmoniously into the suburban Hillsboro community that surrounds it. The entire campus occupies a single block in the Tanasbourne neighborhood, an area known for its shopping malls and apartment complexes. The area is surrounded by high-tech companies and a belt of evergreens—earning this corner of Oregon the name "Silicon Forest."

At the heart of the campus, a tiered outdoor plaza slopes gently upward from the street to the campus's main entrance—a two-story glass rotunda that connects the hospital to a café and adjoining outpatient medical offices. A covered walkway stretches from the rotunda to the public transit stops on the north end of the block, the site chosen for the hospital's weekly farmers' market. Paved walkways wind through dry creek beds and thick native gardens, inviting visitors to crisscross the campus. A circular driveway allows drivers to drop patients at the hospital's main entrance and continue into the covered parking ramp in a single, compact loop. Even the parking structure, which at 90 feet is Hillsboro's tallest building, is a good neighbor. The eight-story structure is covered with giant vertical gardens that will eventually drape its brick exterior with mossy green succulents fed by a rainwater irrigation system.

The same attention to beauty and detail carries on inside the buildings. Surfaces are made of white solid surface material instead of plastic laminate, which is subject to delamination and chipping over time. Nurses' stations are paneled in dark wood, and patient room doors are flanked by nature scenes on floor-to-ceiling panels. Art, ranging from photographic murals to a wall of colorful skateboards, is used to create a healing environment that reflects local culture.

The Kaiser Permanente Westside Medical Center represents the latest thinking in hospital design, which includes not only sustainability, as evidenced by its LEED Gold status, but also design standards that seek to build brand and business values into our hospitals. What I found most remarkable when I visited, though, was what was missing.

With furniture still wrapped in plastic and floors still covered with protective cardboard, there was no toxic off-gassing, no "new car" smell one might expect in a brand new, unoccupied building. With the spring afternoon light flooding in, the hospital felt tranquil and pristine. It was easy to imagine the pleasure of working in such a beautiful environment.

A few months later, when it opened in August 2013, Westside became Kaiser Permanente's thirty-eighth hospital, and the nineteenth built since the early 2000s, when Kaiser Permanente started on a construction program that some have called the most ambitious in recent health care history.

AN EARTHQUAKE'S GREEN AFTERSHOCKS

Prior to the 2001 groundbreaking of Kaiser Permanente's Santa Clara (California) Medical Center, the company had not built a new hospital in almost a decade. And in the meantime, the health care construction industry had changed dramatically, thanks principally to the safety-related aftershocks of the deadly and costly 1994 Northridge earthquake in Los Angeles.

In response to the earthquake, the state legislature passed Senate Bill 1953, giving hospitals until 2013 to meet tough seismic safety goals that would ensure they would remain standing and operational after a large earthquake. A series of later amendments extended the deadline to 2015 and to as late as 2030 for some hospitals. The law required more than half the state's 470 hospitals at the time to retrofit, rebuild, or close their buildings, generating an unprecedented wave of hospital construction in the state at an estimated cost of some $41 billion.[1]

This surge in hospital construction was not confined to California, though the pace was slower and the drivers were different outside the state. Nationally, annual construction survey data indicated costs for construction of acute care hospitals rose by close to 50 percent from 2000 to 2004, and costs for construction that broke ground or were in the design phase in 2004 were similarly running nearly 50 percent ahead of 2000.[2]

All this construction activity coincided fortuitously with an expanding awareness of green buildings and healthy materials in the health care industry, along with a budding assumption that hospital design could heavily influence clinical outcomes and patients' well-being. Not only did the earthquake safety mandates and other forces driving new construction provide a platform for hospitals to put the emerging thinking into play, but they also positioned Kaiser Permanente and other large and expanding systems to push manufacturers to come up with healthier building products.

Kaiser Permanente's first seismic-replacement hospitals opened in 2007 in Santa Clara, West Los Angeles, and the Harbor City community of Los Angeles. But planning and design for these buildings began in the late 1990s, right around the time Health Care Without Harm and the

Healthy Building Network were getting started and the Center for Health Design was expanding. These nonprofit organizations did the early work to educate health care executives about healthier building practices and to introduce design innovations that could improve patient and staff satisfaction, medical outcomes, safety, efficiency, and financial performance.

Their influence is apparent in the earliest of our seismic-replacement hospitals. Our first wave of replacement hospitals opened with nearly all private patient rooms, outdoor gardens to provide views of nature, and abundant windows to let in natural light and reduce energy costs. Hospital furnishings and fixtures used fewer toxic chemicals. Carpets were free of PVC and were backed with recycled safety film from car windshields. Rubber floors replaced vinyl in many of the buildings, and we used paints with no or low levels of volatile organic compounds (VOCs), which were being linked to respiratory illnesses and memory impairment.

These were the early building blocks of what are now widespread practices in the industry.

The Early Champions of Green Building

As earlier chapters note, the pioneers of progress in many areas of the sustainable health care movement often came from outside the health care industry. One of the early trailblazers in sustainable health care design is architect Robin Guenther, now a principal at Perkins +Will, a national design firm. She began challenging the traditional choice of materials used in health care interiors while designing high-end clinical renovations for New York hospital and outpatient facilities in the mid-1990s.

"I began questioning the institutional aesthetic and underlying health issues of using materials with PVC in a hospital setting," recalls Guenther, who used cork flooring to replace vinyl composition tile in an ambulatory care center she was renovating in the late 1990s. Other materials she opted for that had no PVC included raw concrete polished flooring, and tinted plaster paint finishes instead of plastic wall coverings.

"No one talked about replacing vinyl for health reasons at the time," she says. "Colleagues would ask me, 'Why do you want to risk your design reputation on the edginess of the materials you use as replacements for what everyone else is using?' I answered that while it might be risky to be the first to specify something new, it was downright terrifying to be the last one recommending an unhealthy, problematic material to health care owners. Just think about asbestos!" Guenther knew of the work Health Care Without Harm was pursuing to get hospitals to eliminate mercury from their premises, and she figured they would eventually turn to the problems of hazardous substances in building materials. She began meeting with HCWH founder Gary Cohen, Healthy Building Network's Bill Walsh, and others to discuss ways to alert the industry and other architects and designers that there were some materials that had no business showing up in hospital construction.

Guenther had learned early on in her work with health care executives the importance of connecting the dots between sustainability and health and safety. Early resistance from hospital administrators who did not initially embrace sustainable design ideas often occurred because of their inability to see a connection between those disparate issues, she says.

One event that started the early momentum toward cleaning up building materials was the Setting Health Care's Environmental Agenda (SHEA) conference in San Francisco in 2000 (discussed in Chapter 1). "It was a landmark moment," Guenther says. "No one in health care had ever gathered like that to talk about health care and the environment." Health care leaders left the SHEA conference energized with a new perspective that combined environmentalism and healing. In fact, the conference started the momentum for HCWH's first annual CleanMed conference the following year.

One SHEA conference paper that created a stir was presented by Gail Vittori, co-director of the Center for Maximum Potential Building Systems in Austin, Texas. A green building practitioner and environmentalist, she had been involved in projects that laid the groundwork of green building design, including conceiving the framework for the Austin Green Building Program in the 1980s, and the high-profile "Greening of the Pentagon" renovation in the late 1990s–2000s. But Vittori had little experience with health care before attending the founding meeting of the Healthy Building Network in California in 2000, and several months later the SHEA conference, where she advocated the need for "green and healthy buildings for the health care industry."

Architects and health care professionals had long been interested in sustainability, but it was mostly thought of as an environmental issue. It was not until the 1990s that we began to link environmental stewardship to human health, which seems remarkable today, given how obvious that connection is. Vittori took the connection even further by asserting that sustainable design and green building practices should be fundamental to hospitals and other health care facilities as an extension of the industry's "first, do no harm" principle.

"I was stunned to realize that having worked in green buildings for twenty years, I didn't know anyone who had applied a green way of thinking about building design to health care," she recalls. "At the time I thought: 'How have we been so completely missing the sector that should be the poster child for green building?'"

In a paper presented at the second CleanMed conference in 2002, Vittori advocated for a lifecycle approach to facilities, merging capital and operations costs into a single budget to break owners from their strong tendency to focus only on initial costs when making building decisions. Hospital owners and providers, she wrote, "must learn that budgeting needs to change from first-cost to full-cost accounting that, for example, extends a conventional balance sheet to include a value for health impacts and the environment. They must grasp the concept of preventive maintenance and integrated anticipatory design. And finally, they must embrace the concept of partnering with their suppliers and design professionals to continue to explore the linkages between the nature of the physical environment and the impact the environment—including the built environment—has on medical outcomes, user satisfaction, and productivity."[3]

Today, that approach is what the business world calls the "triple bottom line," (discussed in Chapter 3) measuring something not only by its economic value but also by its effect on people and the environment. It is a concept that continues to dominate the conversation among facilities managers.

Vittori did something else that caught people's attention. She extended the existing concern among health care professionals over potentially hazardous chemicals in medical equipment, such as PVC in IV bags and tubing, to concern over the very fabric of the buildings themselves as potentially serious offenders to public and environmental health. She urged the health care industry to use PVC-free flooring, wall coverings, carpet backing, ceiling tile, and plumbing pipe. She advocated for paints and finishes with zero or very little VOCs, and formaldehyde-free wood products.

She also encouraged the industry to contract with design and construction professionals with established credentials in green and healthy buildings, and to train their own facilities staff to operate and maintain their newly green hospitals after they open.

Some of the changes Guenther and Vittori championed began to occur relatively early, but others, including the need for well-trained facilities staff, involved longer term cultural changes.

Starting in 2010, Kaiser Permanente has augmented its facilities design staff of architects and interior designers with LEED-accredited design engineers who can design sustainable mechanical, electrical, and plumbing (MEP) systems into our hospitals, and to challenge the conventional thinking of our contract design engineers. Recognizing that it is not enough to build green buildings, we are also training our chief engineers to run these complicated systems efficiently. Building engineers need a very different skill set than they did in the past. Three hundred of our facilities staff have taken LEED Green Associate classes, and another 50 have completed certified energy manager training through the Association of Energy Engineers in the past year. And we continue to push—and pay for—our employees to earn these credentials. As John Kouletsis, our vice president of facilities planning and design at Kaiser Permanente, puts it: "Healthy buildings are high-efficiency buildings, and they're more complicated to run."

It may have taken us close to a decade to heed Guenther's and Vittori's advice on taking a more holistic, long-term view of our facilities' performance, but their influence on sustainable design and green building materials has served the health care sector well from those first seismic-replacement hospitals to this very day.

TOOLS FOR BUILDING OUT THE GREEN VISION

The enthusiasm with which participants left the SHEA conference on that fall day in 2000 was quickly tempered by the sobering reality we faced back at our offices. We had been trying to understand how to eliminate toxins from medical products, and now we were rightfully tasked with getting toxins out of our building materials as well, but with very little information on how to do it. While sustainable design was gaining momentum in the general commercial building market, health care lagged behind. It was not until the American Society of Healthcare Engineering (ASHE) released its Green Healthcare Construction Guidance Statement in January 2002 that the industry received practical advice on integrating green principles into the design process.[4]

Originally written to help an ASHE subcommittee judge applicants for a sustainable building category in its annual Vista awards, the Guidance Statement established protecting the health of patients and staff (building occupants), surrounding communities, and the global environment as key principles of green building design, and it suggested numerous ways for turning those principles into concrete realities in 10 areas of hospital design. These included integrated design (a collaborative process involving designers, users, construction managers, contractors, and facilities managers), site selection (such as remediated brownfields and proximity to public transit), water and energy conservation, indoor environmental quality, building materials and products, construction practices, commissioning, operations and maintenance, and innovation. Notably, Guenther and Vittori, and Health Care Without Harm's Tracey Easthope and Healthy Building Network's Tom Lent were among the dozen or so members of the ASHE subcommittee that created the Guidance Statement.

Within months of the release of the Statement, Kaiser Permanente leadership adopted the organization's official Position Statement on Green Buildings, in which we expressed our aspiration to "limit adverse impacts upon the environment resulting from the siting, construction, and operations of our facilities," among other things. At about the same time, using the ASHE statement as a foundation, Carol Antle, then Kaiser Permanente's vice president of capital construction, and I worked to develop what we called our Eco Toolkit. It was a lengthy checklist of sustainable design suggestions for use by our project directors in carrying out our multiyear, multibillion-dollar seismic-replacement program. Like the LEED system, it awarded points for such things as environmentally sensitive site selection, recycling construction waste, orienting buildings to maximize daylighting and views, and for general innovation. It was the first time we had ever put something like this in the hands of our project directors and said, "Here, this is what we expect of you."

Not all our project directors embraced it enthusiastically because, understandably, they did not want to risk jeopardizing the cost or schedule of their projects. Nonetheless, it gave us a platform to have important discussions with the community of external architects and engineers we worked with, as well as with our own teams and executives.

A year after we introduced the Eco Toolkit internally, Kaiser Permanente hosted the California Sustainable Hospitals Forum in Oakland. We held it jointly with Dignity Health, Health Care Without Harm, the Healthy Building Network, and the Center for Environmental Health. We invited architects and contractors and gave them the opportunity to interact with some of the leading thinkers in green design. We covered evidence-based energy conservation strategies and the importance of a light-filled, nontoxic indoor environment to patient wellness and healing, things that many of the guests had not considered. We also gave them our Eco Toolkit as a resource and encouraged them to incorporate the strategies into their own projects. But again, not everyone reacted positively. There was resistance on every level. Some of our contractors complained that they had to do more time-consuming research to find new products and different methods for doing things. And we had to battle the persistent and widespread perception that green buildings cost more than traditional ones—a notion that was soundly challenged by the "Fable hospital" analysis in 2004 (discussed in Chapter 3). That landmark work was an early attempt to analyze the economic impact of designing and building an optimal hospital facility. It showed that carefully selected design innovations, though they may cost more initially, could return the incremental investment in a short time by reducing operating costs and increasing revenues.[5] (It was followed up 6 years later by a series of essays known as "Fable 2.0," which updated and strengthened the evidence for the analysis.[6])

But, despite the resistance, there were also early adopters, most of whom have since become models of successful innovation in sustainability (see Box 8.1).

Box 8.1 GETTING RID OF POLYVINYL CHLORIDE IN HOSPITAL BUILDING MATERIALS

Among the early challenges Kaiser Permanente put to its building materials suppliers was a request to come up with a viable alternative to polyvinyl chloride (PVC) in its hand and crash rails and other hospital products. PVC is a widely used plastic that sometimes contains DEHP and other phthalate plasticizers associated with human and environmental health concerns (see Chapter 1), as well as a source of highly toxic dioxins when incinerated. Kaiser Permanente gave its existing building material suppliers 1 year to find an alternative or possibly lose its contract.

Fortunately, one supplier, Construction Specialties, was already in the process of examining whether their product line included any hazardous or harmful materials, recalled Howard Williams, vice president and general manager of the Pennsylvania division. "We were already predisposed to looking for safe materials, but we also knew that Kaiser Permanente was a customer we didn't want to lose. We had a contract that was worth as much as $750,000 a year, and the future value was potentially even greater because Kaiser Permanente had big building plans." What's more, he added, "We realized the move to non-PVC products would position us for the market changes we kept hearing were coming."

Confident in its buying power, Kaiser Permanente upped the ante by telling the company it could not charge more for the PVC-free hand and crash rails and other products it would produce.

Finding a satisfactory alternative to PVC at a low manufacturing cost was no small task. The material Construction Specialties first came up with was 75 percent more expensive than PVC, and it would require the company to spend money to reconfigure its production plant to process it.

The product the firm ultimately offered was a polycarbonate plastic blend resin that was sourced in Germany and produced as a final product in its US plant. In the end, the company invested nearly $2 million in both capital and other soft costs to create the product for Kaiser Permanente.

In the long run, it was a wise investment. "Kaiser Permanente actually did us a favor because by 2007 the market began asking for non-PVC building products," Williams recalled.

Soon, Dignity Health also converted to the new and improved hand and crash rails and other hospital products, prompting additional health care systems to investigate the products. In 2009, Construction Specialties decided to eliminate PVC from all of its wall protection products for all industries.

"You can't be double-minded about this," asserts Williams. "Either you believe in what you're doing or you don't." Williams takes comfort in the fact that more architects and forward-thinking health care organizations are beginning to see the bigger, healthier picture. "They realize you can take an inanimate building and you can make it an animate partner in providing health care," he says. "It's great to know that our materials aren't detracting from the health care being provided within the buildings."

Green Guide for Health Care: First Health Care Hospital-Specific
Building Guide

With demand growing for practical, specific building performance metrics for health care, the *Green Guide for Health Care* appeared in November
2003 as the first sustainable design toolkit integrating enhanced environmental health principles and practices into the planning, design, construction, operations, and maintenance of hospitals and other health
care facilities.[7] Convened by the Center for Maximum Potential Building
Systems (Gail Vittori's organization), in collaboration with Health Care
Without Harm and the Healthy Building Network, the *Green Guide for
Health Care* represented the best thinking from the architectural, environmental health, and health care worlds.

The Green Guide borrowed its organizational framework from the US
Green Building Council's LEED for New Construction system with per-
mission, which was initially released in 1998 but was oriented toward commercial construction and had proved difficult to apply to hospitals, which
have the unique challenges of operating 24/7, employing highly specialized
medical technology and staff, and operating under strict regulatory requirements. The *Green Guide for Health Care*, which customized credit strategies
to be more relevant to health facilities, was created as a catalyst for spreading
green building practices and principles across the health care industry until
such time as LEED came up with a rating system specific to health care.

Building on LEED for New Construction and the ASHE Guidance
Statement, the *Green Guide for Health Care* developed a rating system to
assign credit points for specific features spanning design, construction,
and operations, but because the green building movement was still new to
the health care sector, it was set up as a free self-certifying tool for project
teams to gauge the sustainability of their projects and to make improvements. There were no minimum achievement thresholds or third-party
certifications awarded. But drawing from the best sources in the business,
it gave hospital leaders everywhere a cohesive framework for green and
sustainable design. And by identifying the health concerns each green feature addressed, it enabled proponents to make a stronger business case

for their design choices when they met with resistance from their hospital board members or top-level executives.

Although there was still resistance to the *Green Guide for Health Care* from certain sectors, notably the vinyl and chemicals industries (see Box 8.2), it caught on fast with those who mattered most. Within 4 years of its initial publication—led by Vittori, Guenther, Lent, and a dedicated staff and steering committee—it had been used on more than 119 hospital construction projects nationwide, representing more than 30 million square feet of construction and had garnered more than 20,000 registrants from around the world.[8] A McGraw Hill Construction study published around the same time showed an increasing trend toward building green health care facilities.[9] The percentage of health care executives who said they were "very" committed to green building rose from 4 percent in 2006 to 19 percent in 2008. Nearly 50 percent of the executives who responded to the survey said they believed patients recovered faster in green buildings. No longer were green building advocates just a niche group of starry-eyed hospital leaders, environmentalists, and early adopters talking about sustainable design and linking it to health. Healthy hospitals were officially on the map, and green building practices globally were fast on the way to becoming a business imperative driven as much by client and market demand as by "doing the right thing."

Box 8.2   TURNING THE SPOTLIGHT ON CHEMICALS

The *Green Guide for Health Care*'s suggestion that hospital architects and engineers should avoid a specific starter list of chemicals and formulations was not well received by the product manufacturers and the chemicals industry. The *Green Guide for Health Care*'s list included PVC, mercury, formaldehyde, phthalate plasticizers, halogenated polybrominated diphenyl ethers (PBDEs) in flame retardants, polycarbonate, perfluorooctanoic acid (PFOAs) used to produce stain protection treatments, volatile organic compounds (VOCs), and more.

Listing chemicals to be avoided was one thing. Finding out what chemicals lurked in what products—and then revealing the presence of those chemicals—was quite another. When Tom Lent from the Healthy Building Network, serving as co-coordinator of the *Green Guide for Health Care*, asked manufacturers to share information about the chemical content of their products, many asked him to sign nondisclosure agreements so he could not reveal what he learned. Others told him they did not want to divulge their "secret sauce." "What they really wanted was to keep this information from the end user," says Lent.

Manufacturers challenged the list of chemicals to be avoided, arguing that their products had been used in hospitals for years. The Vinyl Institute, a trade group representing vinyl manufacturers, responded by sponsoring its own self-certification tool, Green Globes. Run by the Green Building Initiative, a nonprofit whose members and supporters include The Dow Chemical Company, The Vinyl Institute, The American Chemistry Council, and the Plastic Pipe & Fittings Association, the Green Globes does not include credits for avoiding chemicals of concern.

To overcome the barriers around ingredient disclosure, Walsh and Lent initiated the Pharos Project, a database that tracks chemicals or other toxic substances used in the fabrication of building materials.[10] Operated by the Healthy Building Network, Pharos started with a specific list of chemicals identified by multiple scientific bodies and federal agencies to have high associations with cancer, reproductive toxicity, asthma, and other health problems. It then focused on researching which finished products in building interiors contained those chemicals.

The first products it investigated included resilient flooring (such as rubber), ceiling tiles, paints, furnishings, hand and crash rails, and wall armor. In hospitals, wall protection systems include corner guards and plastic panels on walls to minimize damage from gurneys pushed along the hallways.

Some of the early findings were disturbing. "We started looking for products that had PVC," Lent recalls. "Hospitals already knew there was a problem with PVC in IV bags and tubing, but we were shocked to learn that 75 percent of global PVC production was going into all sorts of building materials."

Pharos expanded its database as the program grew in sophistication. It also expanded its scope to score products (and their manufacturers) in other environmental and health categories, including the sustainability of wood and plant-based materials and how much renewable energy is used in the manufacturing of specific products.

Pharos gave consumers straightforward information so they would not have to conduct the painstaking research on their own to figure out which carpet or corner guard they should select. With a subscription membership, designers can customize their product search by requesting a list of products that have, for instance, no carcinogens or PVC. As of 2013, the Pharos Project had evaluated more than 1,400 building materials, ranging from giant plastic roofing membranes to additives in paints and adhesives. The most recent products included plywood and engineered wood floors, providing comparisons with other composite woods as well as floorings like carpet, solid wood, and resilient flooring.

"What initially looks like a downer because of all the information we're gathering about chemicals of concern in products is actually great news because it's shining a light on what we can do to avoid those chemicals," says Lent, whose sister died of cancer diagnosed in her early forties.

Another catalogue bringing greater transparency to the building industry is Perkins+Will's Precautionary List, a simple online tool that lists a number of substances that the firm, where Robin Guenther is principal, has, through compiling market and scientific research, decided it would seek to avoid in building products, or substitute with safer alternatives.[11] The website is open to anyone and allows users to search by specific substances, by categories, and by health effects. It is joined by a growing number of hazard lists, including the Living Building Challenge Red List, the Environmental Protection Agency's Chemicals of Concern list, and others.

LEED for Health Care

The *Green Guide for Health Care* rating system was considered by many health systems, including Kaiser Permanente, to be a useful alternative to the more established LEED certification system until, in due course, the US Green Building Council (USGBC) could create a LEED rating that was specific to the unique needs of health care. That course turned out to take a long detour due to deep divisions over the issue of whether the LEED for Healthcare system should offer credits for avoiding certain chemicals in building materials. When the Council finally released the LEED for Healthcare rating system in 2011, 4 years after its initial public comment period and close to a decade following the *Green Guide for Health Care*, it did include credits for eliminating heavy metals and other persistent bioaccumulative toxins in all health care applications. The balance of the groundbreaking material health credits was placed in a Pilot credit library.

More recently, the USGBC has taken the position that the evidence is strong enough to add credits for requiring ingredient disclosure as well as avoiding certain chemicals to the more widely used LEED tool used in mainstream, non–health care buildings.[12] An updated LEED rating system, known as LEED Version 4 (v4), was approved in July 2013 that includes credits for demonstrating manufacturer chemical and material disclosure as well as for building teams that avoid use of certain materials that are linked to cancer, birth defects, and other health or environmental impairments.

In response, a coalition of chemical users and manufacturers led by the American Chemical Council has launched a new "American High-Performance Buildings Coalition" to lobby Congress to stop the federal government from using the LEED program for government buildings, arguing that LEED v4 is not science based and will hurt the US economy and manufacturers.[13]

The ongoing debate over LEED v4's credits for avoiding certain chemicals of concern is unfortunate for many reasons, especially because it detracts from success achieved by the LEED system's rigorous strategies for such things as sustainable site development, water and energy efficiency, and indoor environmental quality, among other things. Those factors accounted for the fact that more than 230 health care facilities had been certified under various LEED rating systems prior to the introduction of LEED for Healthcare in 2011, beginning with Boulder Community Foothills Hospital in 2003. Since then, a number of hospitals, outpatient, and mixed use medical buildings have earned LEED Platinum—the highest possible rating. They include the Kiowa County Memorial Hospital in Greensburg, Kansas; Dell Children's Medical Center of Central Texas in Austin, Texas; and the Oregon Health and Sciences University's Center for Health & Healing in Portland, Oregon.

In April 2013, Group Health Cooperative's new medical office building in Puyallup, Washington, became the first in the nation to earn a rating under the new LEED for Healthcare certification, achieving LEED-HC Gold.[14] In July, the W. H. and Elaine McCarty South Tower of Dell Children's in Austin, Texas earned the first-ever LEED-HC Platinum designation.[15]

LEED is the future at Kaiser Permanente as well. In 2012, the senior vice president for facilities, Don Orndoff, shepherded through a policy to require our construction project teams to pursue a minimum of LEED for Healthcare Gold for all new hospitals, and a minimum of LEED for New Construction Gold on all other construction projects over $10 million— effectively all medical offices and major expansions.

After years of leaving the decisions on LEED certification to our facility project directors and local hospital administrators, Orndoff had garnered support from the organization's top leadership to pursue LEED-certified sustainable buildings at every opportunity.

"As our goals around clean energy, reducing greenhouse gas emissions, and sustainable buildings in general have become more formalized, it made sense for us to adopt what is commonly considered the 'gold standard' for green buildings," said Ramé Hemstreet, vice president of operations for Kaiser Permanente's National Facilities Services Department and the organization's chief sustainable resources officer.

That decision was not unanimous. Cost continues to be the biggest factor among those who do not agree with the policy, despite plenty of evidence that green buildings do not cost much more than less sustainable structures.[16] All of the work to earn our Westside hospital in Oregon its LEED for Healthcare Gold credential, for example, cost less than $200,000 (inclusive of Oregon energy rebates)—money that will be recovered in projected energy savings each year. That is a great return on investment.

In any case, expected improvements in health and reduced environmental impacts stemming from meeting the tough LEED for Healthcare criteria trump the goal of a quick return on investment. "We believe the quality of the built environment contributes to better health care outcomes and the productivity of employees," says Orndoff, adding that his department intends to track such outcomes.

Linking Sustainability to Outcome-Based Design

The Center for Health Design is perhaps the world's foremost source for research supporting the idea that design should be pursued to achieve outcomes—actual results in improved health, environmental impacts, and, yes, cost—rather than design for its own sake or design that cannot be shown to achieve specific outcomes. For that to happen, sustainable design must be combined with evidence-based design.

Here is an example of how the two can support one another: Research done in 1984 by architecture professor Roger Ulrich showed that patients recover faster when exposed to daylight and views of nature.[17] But the study never got much traction until the sustainable hospital movement picked up on it around 2000. If you look at hospitals built in the early- to mid-2000s, you see a gradual moving away from the sterile, institutional feel of the past to more comfortable, hospitality-like settings, with soothing, richly colored walls, healing gardens, and natural lighting.

But is anyone gathering the evidence that such amenities are linked to improved health outcomes? Donna Decker, director of the Center's Evidence-Based Design Accreditation and Certification (EDAC) program, tells of the design work done at a hospital in Ohio to reduce infections. When it opened in 2008, the hospital was thought to be among the first in the country to broadly apply evidence-based design strategies in its design and construction. The quantity, location, and design of its hand-washing sinks, for example, were selected to improve compliance and reduce infections. Patient rooms had a stripe built into the floor and up the wall leading to the sink to draw the eye to it and remind staff to wash their hands. Decker said the hospital claimed to have achieved great results in reduction of infections and in its use of acuity adaptable rooms, another key design concept strongly supported by empirical research. But they had not been able to conduct the formal research as planned. Such is the reality for busy architects and owners who quickly move on to a new project as soon as one project is completed and have neither the time nor the rigorous structure to do a postoccupancy evaluation of the efficacy of the design.

To incorporate the step of measuring outcomes into the design process, the Center for Health Design launched its EDAC program in 2009. By early 2013, 1,400 design professionals had earned the accreditation.

Like the Six Sigma program popular in the business and manufacturing worlds, EDAC provides designers with a formula for "designing for solutions," a more rigorous approach to evidence-based design than has hitherto been widely used. Its eight-step process includes having a vision for a project and defining design goals, which are typically around the "three safeties" of patient safety, workplace safety, and environmental safety. Secondly, EDADC-certified designers use research to find design strategies that tie back to their goals and connect with outcomes. Among the other critical steps are creating a business case and, significantly, measuring and reporting results once a project completes.

Combined with LEED accreditation, EDAC certification positions designers to succeed with their business-minded clients, who value savings and business results as much as they do the more altruistic goal of saving the planet.

Beyond "Do No Harm": Regenerative Hospitals

Although LEED for Healthcare and programs like EDAC certification in evidence-based design represent today's high bar in green hospital design and construction, green building trailblazers like Robin Guenther continue to push the envelope. In an influential article in 2009, Guenther went beyond the idea of green hospitals that simply "do no harm" to talk about "regenerative hospitals" that heal and restore, or regenerate, the degraded environments and communities around them.[18] Instead of simply treading lightly on the earth's resources, regenerative hospitals are zero net-energy hospitals that positively contribute to both the human and physical ecosystems, with open campuses and healthful community amenities, including things like organic farmers' markets and yoga classes.

A good, early example of the kind of place Guenther is promoting is the new Spaulding Rehabilitation Hospital in the Charlestown neighborhood of Boston, which opened in April 2013. Spaulding offers 75 percent of the ground floor of its building, as well as all the surrounding outdoor space, to the broader Charlestown community with such things as a public restaurant that also serves residents, as well as a conference center and aquatics center with two therapy pools where the public can take weekend and evening classes. "We'll rehabilitate patients at Spaulding, of course," says John Messervy, director of capital and facility planning at Partners HealthCare, owner of Spaulding. "But conceptually, it's open to the community to use and benefit from the therapeutic processes we'll have there." The hospital will also include a modern gym and a public rooftop garden overlooking Boston Harbor. It was constructed on a remediated industrial brownfield site, includes onsite combined heat and power systems for both energy efficiency and resilience, and has placed all its vital infrastructure on the roof, safe from coastal flooding and projected sea level rise.

Partners HealthCare's first LEED Gold-certified hospital, the Lunder Building at Massachusetts General Hospital, opened in 2011 and was designed with an interior five-story, landscaped atrium visible from 25 percent of the patient rooms. During the day, the atrium, decorated with bamboo and other plants, is flooded with natural light.

"It's an oasis of calm in the midst of chaos for some of our patients and visitors," says Messervy.

Kaiser Permanente is moving in a similar direction, helped along by Guenther and Perkins+Will. The firm, along with partner firm Mazzetti Nash Lipsey Burch, tied with Silicon Valley-based firm Aditazz to win our

"Small Hospital, Big Idea" international design competition in March 2012. The winners were selected from 108 firms that competed to design a small hospital of the future for construction in suburban areas or smaller cities. Some of the design ideas to come out of the contest include civic spaces that blur the boundaries between the community and the traditional hospital setting and bring nature inside with light wells and rooms that are oriented around a large central courtyard. Their winning energy strategy: a hospital powered by harvesting municipal landfill methane, a potent greenhouse gas that is typically torched off or emitted to the atmosphere. The idea of using landfill methane is a concept that has been implemented at Gundersen Health System and is gaining momentum, as it essentially converts an environmental problem to an energy asset. Such hospitals, when built, move beyond carbon neutrality to actually restore damaged ecosystems and biodiversity, and regenerate the necessary conditions for community health.

This, we believe, is the future of the sustainable health care movement for Kaiser Permanente and, we hope, for hospitals and health care systems across the nation.

CASE STUDIES

Dell Children's Medical Center

The design elements of a hospital are a physical representation of a hospital's values. Dell Children's Medical Center of Central Texas has highlighted their commitment to environmental sustainability by being the first LEED Platinum (the highest rating) hospital ever constructed.[19] And their new W. H. and Elaine McCarty South Tower earned the first-ever LEED-HC Platinum designation.

Dell Children's made use of evidence-based design strategies and a focus on creating a healing environment for the patient. The elements included extensive use of daylight and color, especially relevant to their pediatric population. With windows throughout the facility, 80 percent of the building has access to daylight, extending indoors up to 32 feet from an exterior wall.

Another important consideration was the opportunity to positively impact the surrounding community. Dell Children's energy needs are met through a combined heat and power gas turbine district energy systems owned by the local utility and located adjacent to the hospital that is 75 percent more efficient than a coal-fired plant. In addition to meeting the medical center's energy needs, the plant provides power to other buildings located in the 700-acre mixed-use redevelopment project anchored by Dell Children's. Beyond the visible elements, thoughtful choices were made for impacts on indoor air quality. Products were chosen to sharply limit chemical hazards, including avoiding PVC.

In keeping with minimizing adverse construction impacts, many materials were sourced locally, including Texas red sandstone, concrete with high fly ash content, and recycled glass; other products were manufactured with rapidly renewable materials, including cork and natural linoleum. Built on a remediated brownfield site that was a former airport, more than 47,000 tons of asphalt were recycled contributing to 92% diversion of construction and demolition debris from landfills. The building's exterior features a multilevel healing garden built to accommodate a butterfly garden, a floating stone fountain, and a reflecting pool. Native and adapted plants were used throughout the site, and municipally treated reclaimed water is used to irrigate the outdoor landscape.

Group Health Cooperative Puyallup Medical Office Building

In April 2013, Group Health Cooperative's new medical office building in Puyallup, Washington, became the nation's first health care facility to earn a rating under LEED-Healthcare, earning LEED Gold.[20] The building won points unique to the LEED-Healthcare certification related to criteria in both the building's performance and in patient and staff health and safety.

The building also achieved the unique LEED for Healthcare prerequisite and credit for using an integrated project planning and design process involving the developer, architects, contractors, landscapers, engineers, and Group Health administrators and staff. The result of that engaged team approach is a high-performing building with lower operating costs. Savings in energy costs are estimated to be 29 percent less than the LEED baseline.

Credits related to LEED criteria for connection to the natural world included a green roof and a covered patio connected to the staff lounge. Also, a new LEED for Healthcare credit requiring low nitrogen oxide emissions from furnaces and boilers was awarded for a steam generator boiler that provides all the building's hot water while emitting less than half the allowed amount of nitrogen oxide. Credits were also awarded for minimizing persistent bioaccumulative toxins like lead, cadmium, and copper found in building materials.

"Earning the first-ever LEED for Healthcare Gold certification validates our commitment to enhancing the environmental sustainability of Group Health facilities," said Bill Biggs, Vice President, Administrative Services at Group Health. "The health of our patients, employees and communities depends on a healthy environment and we are committed to conducting our operations in an environmentally sensitive manner."[21]

NOTES

1. Charles Meade, Jonathan Kulick, and Richard Hillestad, *Estimating the Compliance Costs for California SB1953* (Oakland: California HealthCare Foundation, April 2002).
2. C. S. Croswell, "2000 Construction and Design Survey," *Modern Healthcare* (March 13, 2001): 23–36; S. Moon, "Construction and Costs Going Up," *Modern Healthcare* (March 7, 2005): 30–38.
3. Gail Vittori, "Green and Healthy Buildings for the Healthcare Industry," paper presented at CleanMed conference, Chicago, October 2002, 6.
4. ASHE, "Green Healthcare Construction Guidance Statement" (January 2002), http://www.healthybuilding.net/healthcare/ASHE_Green_Healthcare_2002.pdf.
5. Leonard L. Berry et al., "The Business Case for Better Buildings," *Frontiers of Health Services Management* 21, no. 1 (fall 2004): 3–24.
6. Blair Sadler et al., "Fable Hospital 2.0: The Business Case for Building Better Health Care Facilities, *The Hastings Center Report* 41, no. 1 (January/February 2011): 1323.
7. Green Guide for Health Care, http://www.gghc.org.
8. Green Guide for Health Care, *Best Practices for Creating High Performance Healing Environments, Version 2.1 Pilot Report* (August 2007), http://www.gghc.org/documents/Reports/GGHC_V2_Pilot_Report.pdf.
9. McGraw Hill Construction Health Care Green Building Smart Market Report (2007).

10. Pharos Project, http://www.pharosproject.net.
11. Perkins+Will's Precautionary List, http://transparency.perkinswill.com.
12. US Green Building Council, "USGBC's LEED v4 Passes Ballot and Will Launch This Fall," press release, July 2, 2013, http://www.usgbc.org/articles/usgbc%E2%80%99s-leed-v4-passes-ballot-and-will-launch-fall.
13. American Chemistry Council, "ACC Tells Oversight Committee Green Building Monopolies Hurt American Competitiveness," news release, July 19, 2012.
14. Elizabeth Powers, "First LEED for Healthcare Certification in the Country Complete," US Green Building Council, April 18, 2013, http://www.usgbc.org/articles/first-leed-healthcare-certification-country-complete.
15. http://www.dellchildrens.net/about_us/news/2013/07/10/dell_childrens_first_in_the_world_to_earn_leed_for_health_care_platinum_designation
16. R. Guenther et al, "LEED Certified Hospitals: Perspectives on Capital Cost Premiums and Operational Benefits," http://www.perkinswill.com/news/study-contradicts-belief-sustainable-hospital-design-costly.html, Sept 2013.
17. Roger S. Ulrich, "View Through a Window May Influence Recovery from Surgery," *Science* 224 (April 27, 1984): 420.
18. Robin Guenther, "Sustainable Architecture for Health: A Mindset Shift," *Health Environments Research and Design Journal*, July 31, 2009, https://www.herdjournal.com/article/sustainable-architecture-health-mindset-shift.
19. "Dell Children's Hospital Gets LEED Platinum," Building Design + Construction, August 11, 2010, http://www.bdcnetwork.com/dell-childrens-hospital-gets-leed-platinum.
20. Powers, "First LEED for Healthcare Certification."
21. Ibid.

9

Measuring and Reporting

Sustainability Gets Sophisticated

From the operating room to the board room, health care delivery operations impact the natural environment in ways both positive and negative. The net effects can be tricky to measure and can be difficult to communicate consistently. To take just one example, a well-designed hospital like Kaiser Permanente's Modesto Medical Center has a parking lot with permeable pavement to reduce storm water runoff, filter pollutants, and recharge groundwater. But what amount of runoff, pollutants, and groundwater are we talking about? And to what extent are the pavement's environmental benefits offset by the cars in the lot that are getting there with the aid of fossil fuels that pollute our air, water, and soil?

Just as we can often find ways to limit dollar costs without sacrificing quality of care, so too can we limit, or mitigate, the environmental costs of health care operations and often transform them into opportunities, like permeable pavement. As I discussed in prior chapters, there are plenty of opportunities for limiting the environmental impacts of health care delivery that can actually improve the quality of care, like using telemedicine and mail-order prescriptions to improve the reach and convenience of health care while reducing car trips to hospitals and clinics. It is important work, and it is important to measure and report it.

Without good measurement, it is impossible to know the effectiveness of environmental interventions, and we would be at a loss to know how to prioritize our programs and identify environmental hotspots where interventions can achieve the greatest impact. Good measuring enables an organization's decision makers to constantly take stock of the costs and benefits of their operations, both within the organization and the communities it serves. It validates accomplishments and identifies shortcomings. And it underpins the credibility and usefulness of public reports that increasingly are expected of large, environmentally impactful organizations, while also serving to spread innovation and help coordinate sector-wide solutions.

GETTING STARTED

In one of my first discussions with Kaiser Permanente's senior vice president for Community Benefit, Research and Health Policy, Dr. Ray Baxter, he shared a vision in which the organization would be "accountable for all of our impacts." That is saying a lot, and we agreed that part of being "accountable" meant credibly improving our environmental performance and publicly reporting our progress in a transparent way. And "all of our impacts" meant not cherry-picking the easiest or most obvious "greening" activities, but rather doing the following:

- Rigorously inventorying the many activities of our organization
- Identifying their corresponding environmental impacts
- Prioritizing our improvement initiatives based on evidence of significance
- Establishing measurable targets for initiatives
- Implementing improvement programs
- Reporting progress to both our own staff and the public

When we first set out to achieve this agenda in 2008, I tapped into the knowledge of an in-house sustainability expert, Joe Bialowitz, who had experience helping large organizations implement environmental management systems based on the ISO 14001 standard. ISO 14001, developed by the International Organization for Standardization, provides a framework for what organizations need to do to systematically identify and control their environmental impacts, and constantly improve their environmental performance. We completed a planning exercise that, borrowing from the ISO 14001 approach, considered all of Kaiser Permanente's activities and known impacts, and using that information we created SMART (specific, measurable, attainable, relevant, and time-bound) targets in the priority areas, where we could have the most impact on five environmental forces that shape human and environmental health:

- Finding safe alternatives to harmful industrial chemicals
- Responding to climate change
- Promoting sustainable farming and food choices
- Reducing, reusing, and recycling to eliminate waste
- Conserving water

What target-setting tools did we settle on, and how have they evolved over the long haul?

Tools for Measuring and Analyzing

Environmental Management Systems

Attaining goals requires having solid measurement and reporting processes in place, including clearly defined roles, responsibilities, plans, and routines. Environmental management systems based on ISO 14001 provide a clear roadmap for any type of organization to describe, analyze, and improve their processes. Many Swedish hospitals use ISO 14001 to structure their environmental programs, but only a handful of US health care organizations, including Affinity Health, have achieved ISO 14001 certification.

Even if they do not apply for certification, any hospital can benefit from using a step-by-step checklist based on the ISO 14001 standard to identify and fill gaps in its current structures for managing environmental performance, before progressing to initiatives that will more directly reduce environmental impacts.

UTILITY BILL PAYMENT SYSTEMS

Around the same time we set about building our environmental management system, our facilities management leaders began to recognize that our utility bills were a serious problem—and an opportunity. "With literally tens of thousands of utility bills to pay each year," says Don King, our vice president of facilities operations, "we were subjecting ourselves to late payment penalties when the inevitable bill fell through the cracks and, even worse, we were sometimes paying significant overcharges due to tariff rates that were listed incorrectly on our billing statements." So Don's team identified a solution that would help us in many critical ways: a utility bill payment company to whom we would direct all of our electricity, gas, water, sewer, and waste bills. "There would be a modest cost to using this company," Don explains, "but the cost would be more than offset by our savings on late payment penalties and incorrect tariff fees, and we would gain a single system of record for our resource usage." The system took several years to implement completely, and it still requires active maintenance as our real estate portfolio changes. But we now have great visibility into our resource usage, and we have run with it, setting measurable targets and implementing improvement initiatives for energy use intensity, greenhouse gas emissions, landfill diversion, and water conservation.

PORTFOLIO MANAGER AND OTHER ENERGY ANALYSIS TOOLS

In addition to capturing data efficiently, utility bill payment systems often offer analysis tools such as basic greenhouse gas emission calculations and graphs that show trending for resource usage and costs. Organizations looking for more advanced analysis capability can import the data from their utility bill payment system into tools that range from the EPA's completely free Portfolio Manager to emerging "freemium" models (you get some basic features for free but pay for additional features) to subscription-based offerings like those included in many of the sustainability management software solutions that are described later in this chapter.

Kaiser Permanente uses the Environmental Protection Agency (EPA) Portfolio Manager, an online tool for measuring and tracking energy and water consumption, as well as greenhouse gas emissions. Some 40 percent of US commercial building space and half of the largest US health care organizations are already benchmarked in Portfolio Manager.[1] We use it to measure and benchmark the energy performance of our facilities according to the US EPA's Energy Star rating system, which rates buildings on a scale of 1 to 100 relative to similar buildings nationwide. An Energy Star rating of 50 indicates that the building performs better in terms of energy consumption than 50 percent of all similar buildings nationwide, while a rating of 75 indicates that the building performs better than 75 percent of all similar buildings. The rating accounts for weather variations as well as changes in the key physical and operating characteristics of each building. A significant influence on a building's Energy Star score is its energy usage per square foot. Once a building earns a score of 75 or greater, it may qualify for the widely recognized Energy Star label, an assurance to consumers that a building or other product meets high energy efficiency standards.

Use of the Energy Star rating system for buildings is particularly useful for identifying which facilities deserve precious investment dollars. In my organization we have found that the best investments come from facilities that have outsized energy bills coupled with relatively low Energy Star ratings. The next logical step is to conduct detailed energy audits of these facilities, followed by targeted energy efficiency investments.

These investments often involve lighting retrofits and other equipment upgrades. New and improved equipment can include not just the machines that use energy, but the machines—such as meters and building management systems—that measure and report energy consumption. Better visibility into energy use can allow facility managers to do real-time energy management, which typically involves the continuous monitoring of energy use data from meters and submeters. Done effectively, this type of monitoring can be integrated with other aspects of energy management to provide greater visibility and control of an organization's entire energy consumption, as well as analytic data for capital and operational planning. Real-time energy management software is already an important multi-billion-dollar industry, growing at the rate of 40 percent a year, with a fast-growing list of innovative vendors.[2] With so much data available from these types of solutions, the most useful and desirable solutions are likely to be the ones that provide intelligent alerting for facility managers to act on the data when unexplained spikes occur in energy use.

Calculating Health Impacts from Energy Use

An easy to use Web-based tool to calculate a facility's energy health impacts is the Energy Impact Calculator from Practice Greenhealth. The tool uses data on power plant emissions from the US EPA, the Department of Energy, and other peer-reviewed sources to estimate and display carbon dioxide, sulphur dioxide, nitrous oxide, and mercury emissions as well as the negative health impacts caused by electricity use. It estimates premature deaths, chronic bronchitis, asthma attacks, emergency room visits, and more by kilowatt hour per year. It also estimates costs associated with medical treatment as well as societal costs.

Measuring Carbon

The EPA Portfolio Manager not only calculates and analyzes building energy use; it also measures a building's greenhouse gas (GHG) emissions from onsite fuel combustion and purchased electricity. For many health care organizations, it makes sense to focus on emissions associated with building energy use because they can be significant and are the easiest to improve. GHG emissions from energy use account for nearly all of our Scope 1 and Scope 2 emissions, which is typical for hospitals. Energy use also accounts for about $200 million in annual spending by Kaiser Permanente, or an estimated $8.5 billion (in 2008) by all US hospitals.[3] So reducing our energy bill is a significant way to create a healthier environment while improving the affordability of health care.

But a hospital's energy-related emissions are not the whole story when it comes to climate impacts. We rely on The Climate Registry's General

Reporting Protocol to determine our emissions quantities from additional sources that include medical gases, refrigerants, and fleet vehicles. Our 2010 emissions inventory was the most comprehensive GHG inventory ever reported publicly by an American health care organization. It encompassed all emissions sources under our operational control. This means it included emissions from all of our building spaces, regardless of whether we own or rent the space. We chose this operational boundary not only because it is a complete snapshot of our real estate portfolio but also because it will reduce uncertainty about fluctuations in emissions quantities that may arise when our ratio of owned to leased spaces fluctuates. Our GHG inventory was enabled largely by the data contained in our utility bill payment system. It was also based on reports—provided by suppliers and our own purchasers—that detailed the quantities of gases and fuels that we purchased.

As good as our GHG inventory was, however, we still had something to learn from our peers in the UK's National Health Service (NHS). It completed a landmark GHG emissions inventory in 2004 and updated it for 2007, 2010, and 2012. What is unique about the inventory is that the NHS estimated emissions caused not only by building energy use but also by travel and procurement. Surprisingly, these two additional sources—most of which are considered Scope 3 sources of GHG emissions because they are not under an organization's direct control—dwarfed the energy use of their buildings. The NHS emissions inventory demonstrated two facts that many experts were already aware of but had not yet quantified:

- Health care facilities generate massive numbers of vehicle trips by patients, visitors, and employees.
- Health care facilities purchase tremendous amounts of resource-intensive products and services.

Also surprisingly, the most carbon-intensive product utilized for health care turned out to be pharmaceuticals, which are responsible for 21 percent of the NHS total carbon footprint. According to David Pencheon, director of the NHS Sustainable Development Unit, "Our carbon footprint data gave us the information we needed to encourage far-reaching initiatives to reduce emissions associated with travel and procurement throughout the NHS. Some of these initiatives are especially interesting because they can achieve emissions reductions at a lower cost than projects to reduce building energy use. Increasing the efficiency of health care delivery is crucial and a very important first step to cut emissions and save money and other resources. However, the scale of the challenges and opportunities should not be underestimated. It will only be through efficiencies and transformational changes that we will really improve health and care within environmental and financial limits in the longer term. This means addressing complete business models of health care—particularly the role of prevention—where our colleagues at Kaiser Permanente have led the way globally."

How did the NHS figure out its Scope 3 emissions? It employed an input-output model of life cycle assessment to estimate carbon intensities and the emissions of purchased products (see Fig. 9.1).

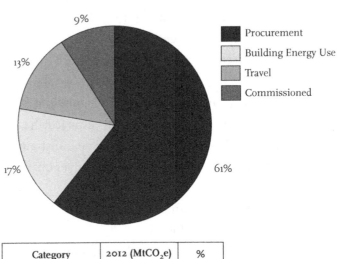

Category	2012 (MtCO$_2$e)	%
Procurement	15.16	61%
Building Energy Use	4.07	17%
Travel	3.15	13%
Commissioned	2.29	9%

Figure 9.1
The 2012 National Health Service carbon footprint breakdown.
(SOURCE: http://www.sduhealth.org.uk/documents/Carbon_Footprint_summary_NHS_update_2013.pdfs)

LIFE CYCLE ASSESSMENT

Life cycle assessment, also known as life cycle analysis (LCA), is a tool for environmental decision support in relation to a product's complete "cradle-to-grave" life cycle (or, if the product is reused, from "cradle to cradle"). An LCA created using your organization's purchasing data allocated to product categories can be a relatively easy way to learn which product categories are responsible for the largest environmental impacts within your supply chain.

Once those hotspots are identified, you can use a more in-depth, process-based LCA to evaluate the environmental performance of one or more products within the categories. A process-based LCA is a time-consuming exercise that is best used for the highest volume products within a supply chain. Nevertheless, the process-based LCA can identify specific areas for improvement by letting you know the degree to which the environment is affected by each phase—raw materials extraction and refining, manufacturing, transportation, storage, use, or disposal—of the life cycle of a product. Based on these results, an organization can compile and prioritize a list of environmental improvement activities.

An important drawback to LCAs is that they do not adequately address comparative risks of industrial chemicals on human health and ecosystems. Comprehensively evaluating human and environmental health impacts of chemicals requires hazard assessment and risk assessment of the substances, something that has been greatly facilitated by the release in 2012 of the BizNGO Guide to Safer Chemicals, which enables firms to track their progress in using safer chemicals (see Chapter 6).[4]

An additional tool for evaluating claims regarding the environmental superiority of one product versus a competing product is the LCA-based Environmental Product Declaration (EPD). The safety science firm UL defines an EPD as a report that documents the ways in which a product, throughout its life cycle, affects the environment. An EPD tells the complete sustainability story of a product in a single, written report.[5] A typical EPD states a product's total emissions of GHGs, ozone-depleting gases, acidification gases, gases that contribute to ground-level ozone, and emissions to water that contribute to oxygen depletion. Other relevant metrics, such as water consumption and impacts on human health and eco-toxicity, may also be included in an EPD.

A recent development that will likely encourage the development of EPDs is that the US Green Building Council's Leadership in Energy and Environmental Design (LEED) criteria now includes a pilot credit that recognizes materials that have third-party verified EPDs. In no industry are these comparisons more important than in health care. Purchasers of building materials and other products in health care organizations should therefore request or require EPDs whenever possible.

MEASURING TOGETHER THROUGH THE HEALTHIER HOSPITALS INITIATIVE

No matter what a hospital currently measures, it should consider aligning its metrics with those of the Healthier Hospitals Initiative (HHI). As discussed in previous chapters, HHI provides an easy-to-use mechanism for identifying and tracking carefully chosen SMART targets that allow any health care organization to improve its environmental performance and contribute to the health and safety of patients, staff, and entire communities. Health care organizations take on these targets by accepting at least one of the six "HHI Challenges." Each of the six Challenges targets a broad-based sustainability impact area—engaged environmental health leadership, healthier food, leaner energy, less waste, safer chemicals, or smarter purchasing—by establishing measurable objectives and identifying appropriate metrics for each (see Table 9.1).

Participating health care organizations report regularly on the metrics for every HHI Challenge they have signed on to, contributing to an industry-wide mechanism for tracking and self-reporting sustainability performance data. A three-tier structure used by the HHI Challenges is designed to make them accessible to health care organizations of all sizes and levels of sustainability experience by allowing them to select goals according to their specific capabilities and resources. After meeting an HHI Challenge's baseline requirements (or providing an action plan

TABLE 9.1 HEALTHIER HOSPITAL INITIATIVE'S SIX CHALLENGES FOR
HEALTH SYSTEMS

Challenge	Objective	Menu of Options
Healthier food	Promote healthfulness by increasing access to healthier, more sustainable food choices	▪ Take the Balanced Menus Challenge and reduce meat purchases by 20 percent ▪ Promote healthy beverages ▪ Increase procurement of local and sustainable food
Leaner energy	Reduce energy use to improve organizational performance	▪ Partner with ENERGY STAR® for energy performance tracking and conservation
Less waste	Implement a comprehensive waste management program to minimize financial environmental and safety impacts	▪ Gather baseline data ▪ Recycling ▪ Red bag reduction ▪ Construction and demolition debris recycling
Safer chemicals	Replace products that cause or exacerbate health problems with chemically safer alternatives	▪ Mercury elimination ▪ Green cleaning ▪ DEHP* and PVC* reduction ▪ Healthier interiors
Smarter purchasing	Aggregate the purchasing power of the health care sector to accelerate innovation in the supply chain	▪ Pledge to support the environmentally preferred attributes in the Standardized Environmental Questions for Medical Products Surgical kit reformulation ▪ EPEAT* computer purchase for environmentally preferred products ▪ Single-use device reprocessing
Engaged leadership	Actively engage board, management, and physician leadership in the sustainability agenda	▪ Create an organizational structure ▪ Adopt a sustainability strategic plan ▪ Develop a sustainability budget

*DEHP, di(2-ethylhexyl)phthalate; EPEAT, Electronic Product Environmental Assessment Tool; PVC, polyvinyl chloride.

SOURCE: Healthier Hospitals Initiatives brochure, http://healthierhospitals.org/sites/default/files/IMCE/public_files/Pdfs/hhi-brochure.pdf

to show how they will meet it), participating organizations commit to achieving Level 1, Level 2, or Level 3 goals within the HHI Challenge area within 3 years. Each level has different requirements, which become more complex as organizations move toward Level 3.

As of early 2014, 836 health care organizations have enrolled in HHI. Some of these organizations are just getting started on the path to environmental stewardship and have opted to accept just one of the HHI challenges; others, including Kaiser Permanente and Partners HealthCare, have embraced all six of the challenges issued by the HHI.

ENTERPRISE SUSTAINABILITY MANAGEMENT SOFTWARE TO THE RESCUE

An organization that is just getting started with measurement and reporting typically gathers much of its data onto spreadsheets. This may be fine for small organizations with a limited number of datasets. But when environmental initiatives begin to mature and blossom, it is likely that you will outgrow spreadsheets. Just think of all of the energy use information available in the form of yearly, quarterly, monthly, daily, and even hourly data. Now multiply that by similar frequencies of data collection for water use, GHG emissions, purchasing, and travel. Then multiply all of that by the number of years of historical data you would like to archive and access, and then start to think about how you will identify trends, make forecasts, and set up plans. And we have not even talked about how you will synthesize and communicate this complex data to your many internal and external stakeholders. It quickly adds up to a major task that can cause major headaches if not addressed wisely. Fortunately, there are relatively mature software solutions that can help you to rise to the challenge.

Enterprise sustainability management software (ESMS) solutions have grown in number and sophistication as the availability of "big data" has increased. Their key selling point is that they provide a single system of record that can store environmental performance data in one place rather than on multiple spreadsheets. These systems, which usually exist in "the cloud" as software solutions, can have many advantages over spreadsheets, including the capability to do the following:

- Create powerful dashboards that delight users and catalyze "no-cost" behavior changes by leaders and frontline staff.
- Efficiently obtain ad hoc and/or customized reports and analysis based on intensity factors and/or business unit.
- Reconcile year-to-year datasets after changes in real estate portfolio characteristics.
- Rely on automatically updated emissions factors based on the latest changes in the environmental attributes of energy supplied in different regions.
- Conform to evolving standards and guidelines such as LEED and the Global Reporting Initiative that facilitate benchmarking across facilities and industries.
- Avoid labor-intensive efforts to assure error-free, "audit-grade" data.
- Improve business continuity by housing all environmental performance in a single location accessible to multiple authorized users and backed up on a regular basis.

ESMS solutions are often very adept at managing data related to energy use and GHG emissions. Many of these solutions also contain modules that assist with other important parts of environmental performance improvement, such as life cycle analysis, supplier questionnaire management, and tracking of initiatives. In conversations with software providers, they report that most customers opt to "start small" with a software implementation focused mainly on energy and GHG emissions. But as customers become more comfortable with the software and their environmental programs mature, they may begin to take advantage of the additional ESMS modules in "a la carte" fashion.

Although ESMS can help an organization compare its various facilities to one another, they can also enable an organization to compare its facilities to others in the health care sector. We do this with the help of

Practice Greenhealth's annual *Sustainability Benchmarking Report*. This report, which is based on data provided by hundreds of health care facilities nationwide that have applied for environmental excellence awards, is an invaluable tool for understanding how our environmental programs stack up environmentally and financially against other leading programs.

TO REPORT OR NOT TO REPORT

So you have collected your data, analyzed it, and maybe even acted upon what you have learned. Now what?

A host of benefits can accrue from sharing what you have learned with others. Effective reporting can accomplish the following:

- Catalyze operational and strategic improvements in your organization.
- Attract customers and new talent.
- Satisfy information requests and demands from large customers who are seeking information about the environmental performance of their suppliers' products and services.
- Demonstrate to regulatory bodies, shareholders, and bond investors that your organization controls risks and has a healthy, long-term perspective.

Reports can be tailored to specific audiences:

- **Senior leaders:** "Steering" is a critical function of all senior leaders and requires clear vision. Your leadership team therefore needs data to evaluate progress and correct course as necessary. Some organizations have even tied executive compensation to sustainability performance, which steers the people who do the steering.
- **The board of directors:** Typically, the board has an oversight role in ensuring that a health care organization is fulfilling

its duties, plus a strategic role of advising on long-term direction. Environmental sustainability performance can figure prominently in both roles. It can greatly reduce costs while attracting additional customers and better talent, all of which is important for both short-term and long-term success. And in the bigger picture, environmental sustainability builds more resilience into health care facilities by reducing dependence on natural resources and protecting the ecosystems that provide new cures for diseases and that support life throughout the planet.

- **Employees:** Most health care organizations, especially nonprofits, are mission driven. Their employees put in the effort they do because they know they are working toward a good cause. They will take even more pride in their work if they know about their organization's environmental accomplishments. And positive peer pressure can be generated by sharing data that describe the efforts of one's colleagues. Reporting data in the form of a full-fledged internal benchmarking system can be an effective way to stimulate conformance with best practices. It can be as large as a quality dashboard that shows resource utilization for multiple environmental metrics within a health care system, or it can be as simple as a friendly competition to see which department can save the most energy. But the principle remains the same: No one wants to finish last, and employees will often try hard to join the club of high achievers.

- **Community benefit stakeholders:** The tax-exempt status of many health care organizations means that they have a responsibility to publicly demonstrate that their tax exemption has been earned through performance that is consistent with social objectives. Tax-exempt hospitals are required to submit a Schedule H Form 990 to the Internal Revenue Service that provides information on the organization's mission, programs, and finances, including the costs of any community benefit and community-building activities, and to describe how these activities improved the health of the communities it serves. Some

organizations also publish a stand-alone annual Community
Benefit report. Kaiser Permanente sees environmental
stewardship as an integral part of its Community Benefit program,
so we include our annual environmental report in our annual
Community Benefit report, published both in print and online.

- **The general public:** People increasingly expect that large
  organizations—especially those receiving any public funding,
  such as Medicare reimbursements—should be held to account for
  their performance. This means not only reporting performance
  to the public but also soliciting feedback and even incorporating
  public participation into decision-making processes (e.g., through
  stakeholder advisory councils, rotating community representation on
  supervisory boards, or through well-publicized town hall meetings).

The number of companies electing to issue annual corporate responsibility reports covering environmental, economic, and social impacts has
risen dramatically over the past two decades, since KPMG began their
annual Corporate Responsibility Reporting Survey. The latest survey, in
2011, found that "where CR reporting was once considered an "optional
but nice" activity, it now appears to have become virtually mandatory for
most multinational companies...."[6] And the great majority of the largest companies reporting, according to the survey, are using the Global
Reporting Initiative framework.

GLOBAL REPORTING INITIATIVE

The nonprofit Global Reporting Initiative (GRI), formed by Ceres and
the Tellus Institute with the support of the UN Environment Program
in 1997, promotes economic, environmental, and social sustainability by
providing one of the world's most comprehensive sustainability reporting frameworks, now used by more than 11,000 organizations.[7] Because
a GRI-aligned report is an integrated financial, social, governance, and
environmental report, it allows an organization and its stakeholders to

consider the ways in which performance in each of those areas may have co-benefits and tradeoffs with performance in the other areas. It takes considerable effort to put together the information and analysis necessary for such a report. And, depending on the organization, it can also require a fair amount of fortitude to be transparent with the public about things they are still working to improve. Despite these concerns, however, companies like Johnson & Johnson have found full disclosure has helped them to build goodwill with the community, without negative repercussions. As for the investment required, Johnson & Johnson's vice president of Worldwide Environment, Health & Safety, Brian Boyd, says, "Our Sustainability Reporting is a terrific investment. While it serves a primary goal of communicating progress to external stakeholders, it also drives real improvement with internal business processes."[8]

The first American health care system to issue a comprehensive GRI report was Dignity Health, which issued its first environmental report in 1998 and has issued a GRI report each year since 2004. "Dignity Health is a strong advocate for measuring the quality of care delivered at the nation's hospitals and publicly reporting performance. Doing so helps us all deliver better care and helps patients make informed decisions about the services they receive," says Sister Susan Vickers, the vice president of Community Health for Dignity Health. "Sustainability reporting," she adds, "also plays a vital role in our efforts to increase transparencies and create a culture of rewards and appreciation in our workforce."[9]

Dallas-based Tenet Healthcare is one of the largest investor-owned health care delivery systems in the nation, with 49 hospitals in 10 states and over 57,000 employees. Tenet started reporting on its environmental, economic, and social impacts in 2011, when it released its inaugural Corporate Sustainability Report. The report was developed in accordance with the GRI framework and met Application Level C Guidelines by sharing information in areas such as governance, economic, environmental, and social impacts.

One of the key components of the GRI reporting process is engaging with all of the organization's key stakeholders to identify the issues they view as most relevant and material. As Tenet moved through the GRI reporting process, they discovered it to be not only a tool for developing a sustainability report but also a mechanism for better understanding the needs of their internal and external communities. This allowed them to customize the content of their reports to meet the information needs of these stakeholders, drawing them further into the conversation.

As Tenet experienced, developing this type of dialogue among community members, whether internal or external, can lead to increased goodwill toward the organization as well as improved brand recognition. It also establishes a communication channel that can be used to address any potential issues or concerns in a timely manner, before they have the potential to turn into major problems. This greatly reduces an organization's reputational risk within the community, and the feedback can also be provided to hospital administration and senior decision makers to help shape company strategy and improve performance.[10]

Health care systems with international operations, such as the Cleveland Clinic, have signed on to the United Nations Global Compact, which has reporting requirements of its own. The UN Global Compact is a strategic policy initiative for businesses that are committed to aligning their operations and strategies with 10 universally accepted principles in the areas of human rights, labor, environment, and anticorruption.

TO VERIFY OR NOT TO VERIFY

"Trust but verify" is a saying that applies to public reporting of environmental impacts. To assure senior management, employees, and external stakeholders that environmental performance improvement is being reliably measured, independent verification is essential. To some degree, all organizations have de facto checks and balances for their environmental data because they undergo the following:

- Routine financial audits that may review accounts of resource costs
- Periodic internal audits of management systems
- Inspections by regulators and accreditation bodies

But absolute resource usage is only a small piece of what can be reported. Effective environmental measurement and reporting is based on many additional calculations—and informed estimations. At any step along the way, mistakes can happen. Fuel pumps that can cost someone a few extra pennies are regularly checked for proper calibration. Should we accept any less scrutiny for an entire organization with significant environmental impacts?

Not only can a second set of eyes help to reduce uncertainty, it also improves credibility with all stakeholders. And credibility has become increasingly important as environmental marketing claims have grown exponentially, setting off frequent allegations of "greenwashing," defined as "when a company or organization spends more time and money claiming to be 'green' through advertising and marketing than actually implementing business practices that minimize environmental impacts."[11]

In 2012, the situation necessitated a broad revision of the Federal Trade Commission's (FTC) "Green Guides" (which were last updated in 1998) to help marketers ensure that the claims they make about the environmental attributes of their products are truthful and not deceptive.

Running afoul of the Green Guides can significantly damage a company's reputation and bottom line. Both the FTC and private parties have already sued high-profile companies for false or misleading environmental marketing claims, resulting in costly penalties and adverse publicity.

A good third-party verifier will not only add certainty to what you report but will also do a "materiality assessment" that can address public skepticism that you are underreporting or not disclosing any of the less appealing but important aspects of your environmental performance. Some organizations might shudder at the thought of disclosing potentially embarrassing information, such as the number of hazardous spills they experienced in a given year. However, as Johnson & Johnson and other corporate transparency leaders have learned, the general public typically understands that accidents happen to everyone, and the important thing is that an organization is honest about their faults as well as transparent in the steps they take to reactively address mistakes and proactively ensure that they do not happen again.

There are, of course, some costs to verification. The costs depend mainly on the amount of information that needs to be verified, as well as the degree of assurance sought. A "limited assurance" engagement is less costly than a "reasonable assurance" engagement and less intensive. But there is no one-size-fits-all strategy. Each organization should work out a verification strategy that suits its needs.

In conclusion, measurement and reporting can be a long and sometimes arduous process. It can be important to "remember the why." Why are you doing this in the first place? Your goals may be many, as will the number of acronyms you will need to learn: LCA, EPD, GRI, CDP, EMS, and many more. But the one that matters most, the one that might be the panacea, is DNA: we need to integrate sustainability into the DNA of an organization. We need to implant the green gene into every functional area, from the board room to the operating room. Good data are actionable data that help everyone understand how the pieces of our ecosystem fit together, and how we can all work together to perfect the puzzle.

NOTES

1. Energy Star, "Use Portfolio Manager," http://www.energystar.gov/buildings/facility-owners-and-managers/existing-buildings/use-portfolio-manager.
2. Paul Baier, "Enterprise Smart Grid Framework Demystifies Confusing Energy Management Software Market," GreenGo Post, March 19, 2012, http://greengopost.com/groom-energy-enterprise-smart-grid-framework/.
3. Practice Greenhealth, "How Healthcare Uses Energy," https://practicegreenhealth.org/topics/energy-water-and-climate/energy.
4. BixNGO, "Guide to Safer Chemicals," http://www.bizngo.org/safer-chemicals/guide-to-safer-chemicals.
5. UL, "Environmental Product Declarations," http://www.ul.com/global/eng/pages/offerings/businesses/environment/services/certification/epd/index.jsp.
6. "KPMG International Survey of Corporate Responsibility Reporting Survey 2011," http://www.kpmg.com/PT/pt/IssuesAndInsights/Documents/corporate-responsibility2011.pdf.
7. Ben Tuxworth, "Global Reporting Initiative: A New Framework?" Guardian Sustainable Business Blog, February 22, 2013, http://www.theguardian.com/sustainable-business/global-reporting-initiative-updates.

8. Brian Boyd, e-mail communication with author, November 2013.

9. Catholic Healthcare West, "An Enduring Mission: Social Responsibility Report" (2009), 6.

10. Tiffany Thomas, "A Breakdown of Tenet's Susceptibility Report," Dallas/Ft. Worth Health Care Daily, September 18, 2012, http://healthcare.dmagazine. com/2012/09/18/breakdown-of-tenets-sustainability-report/.

11. Greenwashing Index, "About Greenwashing," http://www.greenwashingindex.com/ about-greenwashing/.

10

Community Benefit and the Determinants of Health

In the opening chapter of this book, I dated the beginnings of the environmental stewardship movement in health care to the mid-1990s and the launch, by Gary Cohen and Charlotte Brody, of Health Care Without Harm (HCWH). While many hospitals and health care organizations, including Kaiser Permanente, supported various kinds of environmental health initiatives before the launch of HCWH, they tended to be isolated, one-off efforts aimed primarily at improving patient and employee health and safety. Such efforts, while a step in the right direction, fell short of what could be called a movement. Health Care Without Harm provided the necessary inspiration, connections, evidence base, and business case to get things moving in a more or less common direction among a handful of the early champions of the greening of health care. Together with its spinoff membership organization, Practice Greenhealth, it remains the first among equals of the many organizations and coalitions now setting the pace and direction of the movement.

However, for Kaiser Permanente, another time stands out as a key turning point in the maturity of our environmental stewardship work, and it is one that continues to exert a profound influence on our understanding and rationale for what we are doing, why we are doing it, and how we do it. It was the fall of 2007 when our environmental stewardship program was reorganized and reauthorized under the leadership of the organization's national Community Benefit department.

Coming under the umbrella of the Community Benefit program may sound like a simple bureaucratic redrawing of the reporting hierarchy. In another organization, it might have been just that. But for us, it meant something much more profound. It meant that our environmental sustainability efforts on greenhouse gas emissions, toxic materials, waste minimization, healthy and sustainably produced food, green buildings, and other objectives would become formally integrated into a vast range of community-focused programs that address the soul and substance of the organization's historic mission to improve the health of our members and the communities we serve. By aligning our various environmental work streams with the Community Benefit department's multiple initiatives—totaling $2 billion a year by 2012—it also helped to more clearly frame our environmental work in the context of community health as opposed to the less specific objective of "saving the planet," however commendable the latter might be. As Dr. Ray Baxter, the senior vice president of Community Benefit, Research and Health Policy put it, the convergence of the environmental and community health work "helped us to make connections among all the various assets we have across the organization"—from clinical expertise in our medical centers to population health initiatives in our communities to our environmental stewardship work inside and outside the hospital walls. "By utilizing all these separate levers of health," says Baxter, "we can create a concentrated focus on what we've all been calling 'total health,' by which we mean going beyond the doctor's office to schools, workplaces, and community environments that have such a big impact on health." Dr. Baxter is a big-picture visionary, and environmental stewardship fits nicely into that picture of total health.

From a practical standpoint, this more holistic conception of the role of environmental stewardship within the context of Community Benefit meant undertaking a reassessment of what we were doing so that our overall environmental agenda could be prioritized and ranked according to how it impacted the health of individuals and communities. In other words, we had to ask ourselves: What is it about climate change, or about chemicals, or about waste or water or facility design and energy use that is most relevant to human health, and especially to the health of our communities. And of those things, what were we best able to impact, given our unique expertise and resources. In some cases, that meant deemphasizing things that some of us wanted to engage in because it was "the right thing to do for the environment" in favor of other priorities that more directly linked to health risks and the promotion of healthy communities. Above all, it meant focusing first on how our own practices as a health care provider were contributing to environmental risks to health, both within our operations and within our surrounding communities. And secondly, it meant focusing on how our internal environmental initiatives could align with and support other departmental initiatives aimed at addressing the broader social and environmental determinants of health at the community level. That includes things like the quality of the built environment, the availability of healthy food in low-income neighborhoods, and clean air and water—all those factors that shape the health of communities and the people who live, work, learn, worship, and play in them.

In short, the merging of environmental stewardship activities into Community Benefit proved to be a vital boon to reinforcing Kaiser Permanente's total health strategy as it applies to the communities we serve.

MOVING UPSTREAM TO HEALTH DETERMINANTS

One of the most significant benefits of the convergence of environmental health and community health activities has been the development of a deeper and broader definition of both terms. For Rachel Carson and other early environmentalists, environmental health used to refer, primarily, to the health impacts of air and water pollution by hazardous chemicals and other materials, including nuclear weapons. With the growth of the environmental stewardship movement in health care, that narrow perspective was expanded to include the inadvertent negative impacts of health care delivery systems on patients and staff and the immediate environment. This included the issues of medical and nonmedical waste, toxic materials and cleaning products, inefficient and polluting energy systems, and wasteful water consumption, among others. Likewise, community health, at least as the term applied to the community benefit departments of nonprofit health care systems, meant primarily the provision of charity care and expanded access to health screenings and primary health care services for vulnerable populations, including Medicaid patients.

Today, both environmental health and community health, while certainly not synonymous, have converged to involve consideration of a long list of upstream health determinants, including local and regional agricultural practices; transportation options; facilities for physical activity to promote wellness and prevent obesity; protection from infectious agents; the multiple, life cycle contributors to climate change; safe building materials and design; and safe, walkable, and bikeable streets and pathways. More broadly speaking, it may also include the social and economic environment, including good schools, health equity, economic development, and much more. Whether these determinants of health are primarily environmental, social, cultural, or economic is beside the point since they interact with one another in such complex ways as to be often indistinguishable.

The WHO Commission on Social Determinants of Health in 2008 defined health determinants as "the circumstances in which people are born, grow up, live, work and age, and the systems put in place to deal with illness."[1] As discussed in Chapter 3, the work by McGinnis and Foege showed that leading causes of death such as cardiovascular disease, diabetes, cancer, and chronic respiratory disease are the result of controllable factors, including tobacco use, poor diet, physical inactivity, and the harmful use of alcohol. They found that personal behaviors account for 40 percent of premature deaths, followed by family history and genetics (30 percent), environmental and social factors (20 percent), and medical care (10 percent).[2]

It is sometimes difficult to establish clear causal links between social and environmental health determinants and health outcomes due to the lengthy causal pathways and various confounding factors involved. However, strong evidence exists regarding direct health impacts in such areas as transportation, food and agriculture, housing, waste, energy, industry, and urbanization, among others.[3]

Take housing, for instance, for which there is a solid evidence base for the positive health impacts of programs that address such environmental determinants as indoor air quality, dampness, housing design, allergens, building materials, chemically treated furniture and carpets, and, of course, homelessness. Similarly, in the area of food and agriculture there is good evidence for the impacts of chemical and energy use; biodiversity; organic production; fertilizer use; use of antibiotics; agricultural waste and runoff; pesticide use; food transport; access and affordability of retail healthy food neighborhood outlets; the impact of fruit and vegetable consumption; and persistent organic pollutants such as dioxins and PCBs (polychlorinated biphenyls) and metals such as lead and mercury.[4]

These are just a smattering of the environmental factors that we know contribute to the health or illness of individuals and communities, and as such they are illustrative of the upstream direction that health care—especially public health—has moved in (see Box 10.1). This is especially so if we are serious about addressing the persistent racial/ethnic and income-related health disparities that mirror the gaps between healthy environments and sick ones, rich environments and poor ones. The medical care sector, focused on the treatment of disease and injury in individuals, is poorly equipped to address these upstream determinants with population health-based remedies that reach beyond the individual patient. At the same time, the health care system cannot afford to provide the ever-increasing levels of individual, acute care treatment that has resulted from ignoring upstream determinants of health. That mission traditionally has fallen to the chronically underfunded public health sector and its community-based allies, who have been joined in more recent years by the philanthropic sector and nonprofit, tax-exempt health systems driven by a more holistic conception of their responsibilities and obligations to their communities.

Box 10.1   LOOKING UPSTREAM AND DOWNSTREAM

What is meant by "upstream" and "downstream" in discussions of health? The man who first used the analogy, epidemiologist John McKinlay, in an address to the American Heart Association in 1974,[5] suggested that health (or the lack thereof) could be viewed as a river, with health care professionals at one end (downstream) so focused on rescuing drowning victims that they could not look "upstream" to see why people were falling into the water. Thus, "downstream" has come to refer to symptomatic, biological, or psychological manifestations of illness in individuals, whereas "upstream" refers to the factors that contribute to the future illness of populations but which are generally unresponsive to medical interventions, such as drugs or surgery.

For example, obesity and diabetes are viewed as "downstream" health conditions that may be causally linked to "midstream" factors like a person's diet or physical activity levels and to various "upstream" social and environmental conditions like poverty; education; availability of healthy, affordable food; agricultural policies; public transit; and childhood exposure to environmental pollutants. These midstream and upstream factors are amenable to preventive, mostly nonmedical, population-based health care interventions through policy changes in the public and private sectors.

DEFINING COMMUNITY BENEFIT

Today, tax-exempt 501(c3) organizations are required to file IRS Form 990 annually. Health care organizations that include licensed hospitals complete Schedule H as part of their tax filing. Part I of Schedule H is used to report Charity Care and Other Community Benefits expenses, and Part II is used to report Community Building activities.

The Catholic Health Association's widely used *Guide for Planning and Reporting Community Benefit* is an invaluable resource for hospitals and health organizations working to understand and comply with the IRS rules. And in August 2013 with Health Care Without Harm, they produced the very helpful *Healing Communities and the Environment, Opportunities for Community Benefit Programs.*

Environmental costs that may be reported as Community Benefit must first meet a set of criteria, which include responding to a demonstrated community need, improving community health, meeting a Community Benefit objective, and not required by legal or professional standards. Examples of Community Benefit expenses may include teaching parents about safe chemicals in the home, conducting unused pharmaceutical recapture programs, and removing toxins from vulnerable populations' housing.

Community Building activities, on the other hand, include environmental activities that do not qualify as Community Benefit but do strengthen a community's ability to address identified community needs, such as support for community coalitions working to improve environmental conditions like air or water quality, and training community members to monitor environmental health hazards.[6]

The IRS instructions for reporting hospitals' 2011 community benefit activities, released in January 2012, stated, for the first time, that "some community building activities may also meet the definition of community benefit"[7] and their costs may be reported as such. Internal environmental improvements can be reported if the activity is "(1) provided for the primary purpose of improving community health; (2) addresses an environmental issue known to affect community health; and (3) is subsidized by the organization at a net loss. Such expenditures may not be reported...if the organization engages in the activity primarily for marketing purposes."

PUBLIC HEALTH POLICY SHOWS THE WAY

Federal, state, and local health agencies are among the greatest champions of population-based approaches to the upstream determinants of community health. They have been moving in that direction for many years, but the momentum gained great force (and funding) with the 2010 passage of the Affordable Care Act (ACA) and related health reforms that underscore the logic of social and environmental health interventions.

The Affordable Care Act's Focus on Environmental Health Determinants

The ACA itself explicitly called on the Secretary of Health and Human Services to establish a National Strategy for Quality Improvement in Health Care that would pursue three broad aims, including improving the overall quality of care, reducing the cost of care, and improving "the health of the U.S. population by supporting proven interventions to address behavioral, social and, environmental determinants of health."[8]

The ACA also created the $12.5 billion Prevention and Public Health Fund and the National Prevention Strategy, which call for the development of broad-based community partnerships to develop and implement strategies for reducing the prevalence of chronic disease through environmental and social changes, including such things as bike paths, farmers' markets, improved air quality, and parks and playgrounds. The National Prevention Strategy calls on health leaders to promote "healthy and safe community environments (including) those with clean air and water, affordable and secure housing, and sustainable and economically vital neighborhoods." Among its priority recommendations are strategies that address the entire spectrum of the environmental determinants of health. "Safe air, land, and water are fundamental to a healthy community environment," it states. "Implementing and enforcing environmental standards and regulations, monitoring pollution levels and human exposures, and considering the risks of pollution in decision making can all improve health and the quality of the environment."[9] It goes on to cite the importance to community health of air quality standards; improved fuel efficiency and use of cleaner fuels; transportation choices that reduce dependency on automobiles; monitoring, detection, and notification of water-related risks to prevent chemical and biological contamination; and research to understand the extent of people's exposure to environmental hazards and the extent of health disparities resulting from exposures.

A good example of such policies in action is the ACA's Community Transformation Grants program, overseen by the Centers for Disease Control and Prevention (CDC). In 2011–2012 it awarded $187 million in grants to more than 100 state and local agencies and community nonprofits to partner with education, business, transportation, and faith-based organizations. Those grants were a down payment on a 5-year commitment of $900 million to implement broad, sustainable community strategies that will reduce health disparities and expand clinical and community preventive services for more than 120 million Americans.[10] The grants are specifically targeted to support local efforts in tobacco-free living, active living and healthy eating, quality clinical and other preventive services, social and emotional wellness, and healthy and safe physical environments. For instance, a $500,000 grant to Akron, Ohio's Austen BioInnovation Institute, a collaboration of hospitals, city health systems, academia, and philanthropies, is supporting creation of an "accountable care community" dedicated to improving "the physical, social, intellectual, emotional, and spiritual health of the community," as well as "changes across the entire spectrum of the determinants of health."[11]

Aligning with Healthy People 2020

Attention to the upstream determinants of health is also central to the Department of Health and Human Services' Healthy People 2020 agenda, launched in 2010. Among its four overarching goals is the creation of "social and physical environments that promote the health of all groups," with specific focus on six areas of high impact: outdoor air quality, surface and groundwater quality, toxic substances and hazardous waste, home and communities, infrastructure and surveillance, and global environmental health.[12] To carry out its 10-year health improvement objectives across a broad range of health conditions, the CDC issues and regularly updates a "Guide to Community Preventive

Services," known as the "Community Guide," that, among other topics, identifies and recommends strategies for improving community health for which there is strong, systematically reviewed empirical evidence. Many of those recommended interventions fall clearly into the IRS's "community-building" category, including efforts that impact the social and built environments, such as improving food access in food deserts, the walkability or bikeability of communities, tobacco use and exposure, personal safety, and environmental improvements.

COMMUNITY BENEFIT MOVING UPSTREAM

These and many other federal programs are likely to drive private-sector health system community engagement strategies in similar directions. The ACA requires all nonprofit hospitals to work with local and regional agencies and community groups to conduct health needs assessments in their communities at least every 3 years (which was already a requirement in some states) and to implement strategies to address those needs in the interim. Those assessments are likely to indicate less need for charity care after 2014, due to the ACA's expansion of health care coverage to millions of previously uninsured Americans. The expansion of health coverage will likely shift the priorities of hospital's community benefit implementation plans toward more preventive, population-based activities that address the root causes of the most common community health disorders. And these health conditions are directly related to such social and environmental determinants as air and water quality, access to healthy foods, housing quality, economic opportunity, and community infrastructure (parks and bike paths) for active living.[13]

Take the example of asthma, which affects nearly 1 in 10 children and 1 in 12 adults in the United States, including 127 million people who live in counties that exceed national air quality standards. Strategies for addressing the health needs of those high-prevalence counties cannot rely on costly medical care alone to create healthy communities.[14] To be effective and affordable, public health professionals argue they must also target such upstream environmental asthma triggers as indoor and outdoor air quality; secondhand tobacco smoke; chemical fumes from building and furniture materials; certain cleaning products; and various allergens, molds, and dust mites.[15]

Prescribing Vacuum Cleaners at Boston Children's Hospital

Consider how Boston's Children's Hospital responded to a 2003 community health needs assessment that identified pediatric asthma as one of several top priorities in the hospital's surrounding communities.[16] Asthma is the most common admitting diagnosis at Children's and at other pediatric hospitals, and 70 percent of Boston Children's asthma-related hospitalizations came from surrounding neighborhoods with large populations of low-income African American or Latino families. The hospital, which already had excellent clinical care programs for asthma, decided in 2005 to provide a more intensive, preventive approach to the problem through a new community outreach program known as the Community Asthma Initiative (CAI).

Using case management nurses and community health workers to provide personalized care plans, the program also conducts personal visits to patients' homes to assess and remediate potential environmental asthma triggers, such as dust, pests, mold, and mildew, which are common in a lot of low-income housing. The remediations include such simple, comparatively inexpensive interventions as providing families in need with vacuum cleaners, mattress encasements, and food containers to prevent rodent and insect contamination. If required, the program will also bring in an integrated pest control service and refer patients to local inspection agencies or legal services to help force landlords to make environmental improvements to their buildings.

An evaluation of the CAI program at the end of 2011 found that the 800 young asthma patients who received home visits experienced 81 percent fewer asthma-related hospitalizations, 62 percent fewer emergency room visits, 41 fewer missed school days, and 46 percent fewer missed work days for parents. The children's health care costs (largely borne by taxpayers) fell by 40 percent.

Similarly impressive community health improvements with high pay-offs in publicly borne health care costs are being realized by nonprofit hospitals' social and environmental community interventions all across the country.[17]

The three-state Dignity Health system created a Community Investment Program that focuses on improving community health through affordable housing, job creation, education, social services, and health services for low-income families. As of June 2012, the program had invested more than $131 million in 219 organizations. In that year, alone, it provided loans for the construction of 16,324 units of housing and 13 nonprofit facilities serving disabled or homeless children, women, families, and seniors.[18]

Dignity made another $2.5 million loan to the California Endowment's FreshWorks Fund to help finance the development of grocery stores and other forms of fresh food retail in underserved communities throughout California.[19] After just 1 year, the Fund, of which Kaiser Permanente is a founding sponsor and major donor, had raised more than $260 million for grants and loans from a variety of public and private partners and had provided critical financing for development of full-service grocery stores and year-round farmers' markets in half a dozen California communities. Two major loans have gone to grocery ventures in West Oakland, a food desert of more than 20,000 residents. One will seed a fundraising campaign to raise as much as $3 million to create a 12,000-square-foot, full-service fresh-food grocery, creating 35 permanent jobs as a co-benefit. Another will help support a worker-owned fresh food store that is the first retail outlet of any kind to offer fresh food in the neighborhood.

Partnerships for Upstream Interventions

This kind of major initiative, providing hundreds of jobs plus local options for healthy eating, cannot happen without multiple partners investing funds, expertise, technical assistance, and other forms of support. For that reason, other health organizations often team up with regional or national public–private partnerships devoted to the sustainable development of healthy communities—coalitions like the Convergence Partnership, the Healthier Hospitals Initiative, and the Partnership for a Healthier America, founded to support First Lady Michelle Obama's "Let's Move" campaign to wipe out childhood obesity within a generation. What the best of these and other community health programs have in common is that they exist at the intersection of environmental health and community health. They address obstacles to community health in ways that make for a healthier planet and healthier people.

The Convergence Partnership, for instance, has brought large, health-oriented public and private funders together to support initiatives and health policy reforms that address the nexus of social and environmental determinants of obesity. Successful advocacy efforts backed by the partnership have included creation of the National Prevention and Wellness Trust, the Community Transformation Grants program, the federal Communities Putting People to Work program, and the $400 million National Healthy Food Financing Initiative, a national version of the California FreshWorks Fund. The coalition has also provided technical and financial support for health-promoting policy changes in the areas of surface transportation, land use planning, and agriculture.

"We try to focus our investments on ways that can change the food and physical activity environment while also reducing carbon dioxide emissions," said Loel Solomon, vice president for community health initiatives in our Community Benefit department. "When we're able to change local land use and transportation plans in ways that get away from sprawl and move toward more compact and mixed use development, we're increasing people's options for walking and biking and using public transit, all of which is good for carbon dioxide reduction and disease prevention. So a lot of the things that we get interested in are at that intersection of the environment, local economic development, and population health. Good solutions solve many problems."[20]

Kaiser Permanente's Community Health Initiatives

At Kaiser Permanente, this search for solutions with multiple benefits is at the heart of the Community Health Initiatives (CHI), which is a major feature of an overall community engagement agenda. The CHI program started around 2003 as prevention-driven, community-based efforts to reverse the obesity epidemic and related diseases. As the program has grown from 3 to 40 communities, with a cumulative 8-year investment of more than $36 million as of 2012, its reach has expanded to address the full panoply of social and environmental factors that contribute to obesity—land use planning; school nutrition programs; neighborhood gardens; public safety; healthy food access; support for local farmers committed to sustainability practices; economic development; and development of parks, playgrounds, bike and hiking paths, and safe streets.

A good example of a CHI community is the Westwood neighborhood of Denver, a low-income community afflicted by high rates of depression, diabetes, obesity, drug addiction, and crime. In 2008, Westwood joined with more than 20 Colorado communities participating in LiveWell Colorado, which public and private funders helped launch in 2006 to promote policy, lifestyle, and environmental changes that support various goals related to the health of the neighborhood and its residents. Since joining the collaborative, Westwood residents have built safe new playgrounds, two community gardens, 87 backyard gardens, and sponsored regular farmers' markets, graffiti cleanups, food classes, and free sports and exercise programs.[21]

"What we've found is that the community gardens, clean and safe walking paths, group exercises programs, and newly built parks and playgrounds got residents out of their homes, talking to one another, and engaging with their neighbors," says Rachel Cleaves, project coordinator for LiveWell Westwood. "And once those relationships were formed, the community became a safer and more enjoyable place to live."[22]

One difficulty of interventions aimed at far upstream health determinants is evaluation and measurement of their impacts. Since the relationship between the interventions, such as building a bike path, and the desired health outcomes, such as reduction in obesity, is indirect and develops over a long period, it can be extremely hard to measure with any accuracy. To address this issue and strengthen the evidence base for these kinds of interventions, Kaiser Permanente worked with the CDC to develop more effective measures for evaluating the efficacy and sustainability of our prevention efforts, resulting in a model the CDC it now using across the nation. We have also used these new evaluation tools to study Kaiser Permanente's own CHI programs and others we have cosponsored with the California Endowment, another major health care philanthropy, and we shared the findings through an entire special issue of the *American Journal of Public Health* (November 2010).[23] Among the findings, our California CHI communities in Santa Rosa, Modesto, and Richmond all saw statistically significant increases in the percent of residents benefiting from walkable neighborhoods, healthier school food policies, development of parks and bike trails, and transportation improvements. In all three communities, neighborhood-level changes reached up to 35 percent of all residents. A subsequent evaluation of the CHI communities in 2013 demonstrated that nearly 600 community change strategies are being implemented in 34 communities encompassing policy, environmental, and programmatic changes as well efforts to build community capacity to make changes in the future. These community changes, two thirds of which have been implemented, will touch 530,000 residents, including 156,000 youth. Combining strategies that target the same health outcome (e.g., minutes of physical activity) into clusters resulted in 98 strategies in community settings and 92 clusters in school settings. In the few cases where both pre- and post-population-level surveys have been conducted, we have found measurable improvements in school-based clusters.[24]

There are many examples of single interventions that health systems can and are pursuing that address multiple social and environmental problems. The Denver B-cycle program offers residents and visitors a viable transportation alternative to cars that serves to increase daily physical activity, save money, reduce reliance on fossil fuels and production of air toxins and carbon emissions, and create local jobs. Supported by a 3-year, $450,000 grant from lead sponsor Kaiser Permanente, the program allows people to purchase short- or long-term memberships that entitle them to pick up and return bikes at numerous stations throughout the city. In less than 3 years, the program logged more than 500,000 rides, leading to an estimated 30 million calories burned and 1.5 million pounds of carbon offset. Surveys show that 35 percent of respondents reported using Denver B-cycle to replace trips totaling 1.5 million miles that otherwise would have been made by car. Denver B-cycle is now integrated into Denver's overall transportation system and represents a critical aspect of Denver Greenpoint, the city's climate change action plan.[25] It also has spurred development of similar bike-sharing programs in cities across the country.

CONCLUSION: IF IT BENEFITS COMMUNITY HEALTH, IT IS WORTH DOING

In the final analysis, most health systems engage with their communities not because they are incented to do so by federal and state tax law, but because they are mission-driven organizations that care deeply about the health of their communities. They know that individuals' health depends on the health of the communities in which they live, work, learn, and play, and that the health of those communities depends on a healthy environment—health-sustaining air, water, soil, and all natural resources. They strongly believe, on the basis of compelling evidence, that when they invest their dollars and their expertise in promoting healthy social and physical environments, they are benefiting their communities and contributing to the health of everyone.

NOTES

1. World Health Organization, *Closing the Gap in a Generation: Health Equity through Action on the Social Determinants of health: Report from the Commission on Social Determinants of Health* (Geneva, Switzerland: WHO, 2008), http://www.who.int/social_determinants/thecommission/finalreport/en/index.html
2. J. Michael McGinnis et al., "The Case for More Active Policy Attention to Health Promotion," *Health Affairs* 21, no. 2 (March 2002): 78–93.

3. See World Health Organization, "The Determinants of Health," http://www.who.int/hia/evidence/doh/en/index.html.

4. Ibid.

5. Marjorie Cypress, "Looking Upstream," *Diabetes Spectrum* 17, no. 4 (November 4, 2004): 249.

6. Julie Trocchio, "How Community Building Aligns with Public Health," *Health Progress* (September–October 2011).

7. Hilltop Institute, "Community Benefit Briefing," March 2012, http://www.hilltopinstitute.org/hcbp_newsletter_2012mar.cfm.

8. National Strategy for Quality Improvement in Health Care, *Report to Congress: Executive Summary* (Washington, DC: US Department of Health and Human Services, March 2011).

9. US Department of Health and Human Services, Office of the Surgeon General, *National Prevention Strategy* (2011), 14.

10. US Centers for Disease Control and Prevention, "Community Transformation Grants," http://www.cdc.gov/communitytransformation.

11. Austen BioInnovation Institute in Akron, "Healthier by Design: Creating Accountable Care Communities" (February 2012), http://www.abiakron.org/Data/Sites/1/pdf/accwhitepaper1211v5final.pdf.

12. HealthyPeople.gov, "HHS Prevention Strategies," http://www.healthypeople.gov/2020/about/prevStrategies.aspx.

13. Martha H. Somerville et al., "Hospital Community Benefits After the ACA: Community Building and the Root Causes of Poor Health," issue brief (Baltimore: Hilltop Institute, University of Maryland, 2012), 4.

14. US Environmental Protection Agency, "Our Nation's Air: Status and Trends Through 2008," http://www.epa.gov/airtrends/2010.

15. Agency for Toxic Substances and Disease Registry, "Environmental Triggers of Asthma," http://www.atsdr.cdc.gov/csem/csem.asp?csem=18.

16. M. Laurie Cammisa and Elizabeth R. Woods, "Boston Children's Hospital's Approach to Community Health: Using Programs to Achieve Systemic Change," February 22, 2013, http://healthyamericans.org/health-issues/prevention_story/boston-childrens-hospitals-approach-to-community-health-using-programs-to-achieve-systemic-change.

17. Somerville, "Hospital Community Benefits," 11.

18. Dignity Health, "Corporate Social Responsibility Report" (2011).

19. Ibid.

20. Loel Solomon, interviewed by Judith Nemes and Jon Stewart.

21. Kaiser Permanente, *LiveWell Colorado: Kaiser Permanente 2011 Community Benefit Report*, 34.

22. Ibid.

23. *American Journal of Public Health* 100, no. 11 (November 2010).

24. A. Cheadle et al., "Kaiser Permanente's HEAL-CHI Obesity-Prevention Initiative in Northern California: Evaluation Findings and Lessons Learned," *American Journal of Health Promotion* (October 2013).

25. https://denver.bcycle.com.

Note: Tables and figures are shown in italics.

Adams, L., 153
Adams, R., 102
Advocate Christ Medical Center, 122
Affinity Health, 217
Affordable Care Act (ACA), 65–66
   community health needs assessments, 245
   focus on environmental health determi-
     nants, 243–244
Agency for Healthcare Research and
    Quality, 73
American Chemical Council, 206
American Chemistry Council, 140, 204
American Hospital Association (AHA),
    19, 107, 115
American Nurses Association, 8, 135
American Society of Healthcare Engineering
    (ASHE), 13, 71, 75–76, 115, 198, 202
Anastas, P., 148
Andrade, R., 119
animal studies, phthalate exposure risks, 2
antibiotic resistance, 89–90
Antle, C., 199
Arrow Value Recovery (formerly
    Redemtech), 125
Association of Energy Engineers, 197
Association for the Healthcare
    Environment (AHE), 115
Association for the Healthcare Resource &
    Materials Management (AHRMM), 115
asthma, 245–246

   pediatric asthma, 246–247
audits of environmental performance,
    232–234
Austen BioInnovation Institute, 244

Baker, R., 177, 179
Balanced Menus challenge, 100
Baxter, R., xii, 62, 216, 237
behavioral and environmental protection
    strategy, 66–67
Bellevue Hospital, 32
benchmarks, 21–23
Berkeley Center for Green Chemistry,
    150–151
beverage purchases, eliminating
    sugar-sweetened (SSBs), 101–103
Bialowitz, J., xii, 40, 41, 217
Biggs, B., 213
bike-sharing programs, 250–251
biomass technology, 45–46, 151
Bio-Plastics Pilot, 150
bisphenol-A (BPA), 92, 135
   in baby food containers, 140
   as endocrine disrupter, 139–140
BizNGO Guide to Safer Chemicals, 223
Boston Children's Hospital, 246–247
bottled water use, 52
Boulder Community Foothills Hospital,
    207
Boyd, B., 231

Breast Cancer Fund, 140
Broadlane, 173, 188
Brody, Charlotte, 5–6, 7, 14, 108, 236
building. *See* hospital design
building engineers, 197
business case for greening of business
    operations, 59
Business NGO Working Group, 143

California Endowment, 247, 250
California Proposition65, 152
California Sustainable Hospitals Forum,
    199
carbon dioxide emissions
    hospitals, 12
    reduction, 38
carbon footprint data, 221
carbon neutrality, 42–43
carpet, PVC-free, 146
Carson, Rachel, 15, 238
Catholic Health Association, 241
CDC (Centers for Disease Control and
    Prevention)
    antibiotic resistance, 89–90
    climate change policy, 35–36
    Community Transformation Grants, 244
    DEHP exposure risks, 2
    environmental stewardship, 64
    "Guide to Community Preventive
        Services,"244–245
    measuring community prevention
        efforts, 250
    National Biomonitoring Program, 11, 135
    prevention/environmental health ap-
        proach, 66
Center for Environmental Health (CEH)
    guidelines for electronics, 188–189
Center for Health Design, 194, 208
    Evidence-Based Design Accreditation and
        Certification (EDAC) program, 208–209
Center for Maximum Potential Building
    Systems, 20, 72
    green building design, 195–196
    sustainable food, 84
Ceres, 17, 36
    Global Reporting Initiative, 230–232

Ceres Principles, 17–18
chemical agents used in hospitals, 13
    See also industrial chemicals; toxic
        chemicals
chemical fertilizers, 88
Chiang, S., 189
chimney sweeps, 132–133
chronic diseases, 64–67
    food system related, 81
    industrial chemical exposure, 132, 134,
        135
    overweight and obesity, 80–81, 86–87
    pesticide exposure, 88
Clancy, C., 73
cleaning products, viii, 147, 157–158
CleanMed conferences, 20, 168, 179, 195,
    196
Cleaves, R., 249
Cleveland Clinic, 47–48, 232
climate change
    air pollution, 34–35
    dimensions of, 26
    epidemiology of, 26–28
    excess heat, 30–31, *31*
    extreme weather events, 31–33
    food system impact, 93
    food-, water-, and insect-borne diseases,
        35
    health care industry impact on, 12
    health care priorities, 37–38
    health-related impacts, 29–30, *30*
    IPCC on, 25
    Kaiser Permanente response, 38–40
    policy response, 35–37
    potential health impacts, 12
    threat to global health, 28–35
The Climate Registry's General Reporting
    Protocol, 220–221
Coates, G. W., 150
Cohen, Gary, 5, 6–7, 14, 21, 108, 169, 195,
    236
Collins, A., 126
Community Asthma Initiative (CAI),
    246–247
community benefit
    defining, 241–242

IRS instructions, 241–242, 245
  moving upstream, 245–248
community health framework, 237–239
  Dignity Health system, 247
  health care missions, 251
  partnerships for upstream interventions,
    247–248
Community Health Initiatives (CHI),
    249–251
community needs assessment
  ACA requirements, 245
  pediatric asthma example, 246–247
community-supported agriculture (CSA)
    programs, 99
Community Transformation Grants
    program, 244, 248
composting, 111
computer purchasing, 49
  controlling waste, 181–182
  energy use, 183
  purchasing strategies for greener
    electronics, 184
  toxic substances, 182
  waste generation, 182–183
concentrated animal feedlot operation
    (CAFO), 89
construction and demolition debris
    (C&D), 111
  recycling, 125–126
construction industry (health care),
    193–194
  green building champions, 194–198
Construction Specialties, 200–201
Consultative Group on International
    Agricultural Research (CGIAR), 93
Convergence Partnership, 248
Corporate Responsibility Report Survey
    (KPMG), 230
Costello, A., 29
Culinary Institute of America (CIA), 80

D'Angelo, J. L., 47–48
Dartmouth-Hitchcock Medical Center, 102
data storage, 50
Decker, D., 208, 209
DEHP (di[2-ethylhexyl] phthalate), 2–4

in food packaging, 92
  Kaiser Permanente policy, 141
  reduction programs, 22
  studies, 4, 135
Dell Children's Center of Central Texas,
    207, 211–212
dengue, 12, 35
Dentzer, S., 8
Denver, 249–251
Denver B-cycle program, 250–251
deRiggi, T., 16–17
design of hospitals. See hospital design
DES for pregnant women, 139
diabetes, 241
Dignity Health (was Catholic Healthcare
    West), 17
  Community Investment Program, 247
  GRI reports, 231
  Guidelines for Environmentally
    Preferable IT Purchasing and
    Management, 187–188
  non-PVC building materials, 201
  purchasing policies, 167, 168
  Social Responsibility Report, 168
  TSCA reform, 155
  energy consumption and GHGs,
    43–44
  hospital garden program, 80
  landfill gas as energy source, 48–49
dioxin
  effect on humans, 114
  EPA warnings, 5
  incineration of medical waste, 6, 114
disposable medical supplies, 121–123
Dominican Hospital, 80

Easthope, T., 198
"Eco-Toolkit," 71, 199
electronic health record systems, 129, 181,
    188
Electronic Product Environmental
    Assessment Tool (EPEAT), 49, 171,
    181
  environmental rating system, 184,
    186–187
  growth of standards, 187

Electronic Product Environmental
    Assessment Tool (EPEAT) (*Cont.*)
  Kaiser Permanente, 187–188
  website, 185
electronics recycling, 124–125
Elkington, J., 59
Emory medical school, 18
energy
  sustainable energy policy, 39
Energy Star, 185
  building ratings, 219
energy use
  analysis tools, 218–220
  calculating health impacts, 220
  of electronic devices, 183
  energy management software, 220
  Portfolio Manager, 219
enterprise sustainability management
    software (ESMS), 226–228
environment
  role in disease, 8
environmental capital, 60
environmental health, 238–239
environmental management systems,
    217–218
environmentally preferable purchasing
    (EPP)
  beginning stages, 145, 167
  Carter administration origins, 166
  case studies, 178
  embedding into organizational DNA,
    176–178
  growth of, 167–168
  Kaiser Permanente, 56, 172–176
  performance review of procurement
    employees, 177
  savings, 178–179
  strategic risk and opportunity
    assessments, 180
Environmental Product Declaration
    (EPD), 223–224
Environmental Protection Agency (EPA)
  agreement with AHA, 19, 107
  dioxin effects, 5
  early focus, 8, 10
  green chemistry, 148, 150

  hazardous waste sites, 137
  Portfolio Manager, 218–219
  toxic chemicals, 10, 136, 154
  US greenhouse gases, 113
environmental stewardship movement
  beginnings, 4–5, 236
  business case for, 64
  environmental health issues, 238–239
  origins of, 14–15
  prevention paradigm, 64–67
  reorganized at Kaiser Permanente, 236–237
environmental sustainability movement
  health care entrance into, 21
  savings achieved, 55–56
Environmental Working Group, 138
e-Stewards® recycling, 125, 185
European Chemicals Agency, 157
European Union, 89
  EPP procurement, 171
  REACH legislation, 156, 157
  Restriction of the use of certain
    Hazardous Substances (RoHS), 184
Evidence-Based Design Accreditation
    and Certification (EDAC) program,
    208–209
Extended Producer Responsibility (EPR)
    Principle, 143

Fable Hospital, 68–70, 200
Farm Bill, 93–94
farmer's markets, 78–79, 95
Federal Trade Commission, 233
flame retardant standards, 152
  halogenated flame retardants (HFRs), 159
  medical furniture, 159
Fletcher Allen Health Care, 18
  healthy food, 80, 91
Foege, 239
Food and Drug Administration (FDA)
  on BPA, 139–140
  disposable devices, 121
  phthalate risks, 2, 4
food hubs and cooperatives, 97–99
FoodMed, 84–85
food packaging
  bisphenol-A (BPA) in, 92

phthalates in, 92
styrene in, 92
Food Safety and Modernization Act (2010), 83
food system
   climate change link, 93
   contaminated products, 83
   healthy hospital initiatives, 94–95
   industrial food system, 82–83, 93
   local grower support, 99
   locally grown, 80
   pesticide and fertilizer residues, 87–88
   policy reforms, 93–94
   purchasing, 52, 180
   steroid and antibiotic use, 89–91, 96
   sugar-sweetened beverages (SSBs), 101–103
   "sustainable," 84
   sustainable food purchasing, 96–97
   sustainable objectives, 94
fossil fuel emissions, 45
Fresh Works Fund, 247, 248
Frieden, T., 90
Frumkin, H., 64

Garfield, S., xi
Geller, M., 108, 127, 128
Gerwig, K., xiii
Gibson, A., 100
GL Envision LLC, 44, 45, 46
Global Reporting Initiative (GRI), 17–18,
   230–232
gloves, viii, 6, 146
Gotto, R., 169
Gould, R. M., 27
green chemistry, 148, 150
   twelve principles, 148–149
Green Chemistry Initiative, 153
Green, D., 42
Green-e, 186
Green-e Energy renewable energy
   certificates (RECs), 41
Green Globes, 204
Greenguard, 186
Green Guide for Health Care, 20
   described, 202–203
   impact of, 72
   LEED for Healthcare, 73

listing chemicals, 203–204
   resistance to, 203
   sustainable food, 84
Green Guides (Federal Trade
   Commission), 233
"Green Healthcare Construction Guidance
   Statement," 71, 198
green health care movement
   growth of, 19
greenhouse effect, 27
greenhouse gas emissions
   inventory reported (2010), 221
   Portfolio Manager for analyzing, 220
   Scope 3 emissions, 221–222
   tools for analyzing, 218–220
greenhouse gases (GHGs)
   anthropogenic sources, 26, 26–28, 27
   Dignity Health commitment, 43–44
   health care sector, 12–13, 37–38
   industrial agriculture, 93
   IPCC reports, 25
   Kaiser Permanente approach, 38–39, 180
   landfill gas as fuel source, 48–49
   past climate changes, 26
   Proposition23, 43
   rates of increase of three major, 28
   reduction strategies, 42
   tools for calculating consumption, 38
   traditional waste disposal, 113
Greening Our Built World, 74
Greening the Supply Chain initiative, 168
green projects
   three objectives, 58–59
Green Revolution, 88
Green Seal, 185–186
green teams, 16, 17
greenwashing, 184–185
Group Health Cooperative, 73, 207, 212–213
group purchasing organizations (GPOs),
   167–168
   data collection, 177
   Kaiser Permanente, 173, 177
   standardizing questions to suppliers,
   168–172
Guenther, R., 194–195, 196, 198, 203, 205,
   209–210

"Guide to Community Preventive Services"
    ("Community Guide"), 244–245
*Guide for Planning and Reporting
    Community Benefit*, 241–242
Gundersen Lutheran Health System, 44–47
    food cooperatives, 97–98
    landfill methane energy source, 211

halogenated flame retardants (HFRs), 159
Halvorson, G., xi, 181
Hanson, D., 29
Harvard Medical School, 18, 123
Harvard School of Public Health, 80
Harvie, J., 84
Hawken, P., 60
hazardous products, 143–144
    See also industrial chemicals; toxic
        chemicals
    flame retardants on furniture, 152
    Green Chemistry Initiative, 153
    hazard lists, 205
    identifying, 145
    state policy, 151–153
    "Targeted Ten" list, 146–147
health care
    bottom line considerations, 61–64
    changing landscape, vii–x
    chemical toxicity, 140–141
    green vanguard, 21
    potential of sector, 14
    savings from sustainable operations, 55
Health Care Without Harm, 4–8
    See also Practice Greenhealth
    Balanced Menus challenge, 100–103
    biomonitoring, 135
    building design initiative, 20, 72, 195
    CleanMed conference, 20
    collaborative strategy, 7
    conference, 70–71
    DEHP in plastics, 2
    early members, 17
    facing environmental health hazards,
        8, 10
    as first among equals, 236
    harmful chemicals, 142

*Healing Communities and the
    Environment, Opportunities for
    Community Benefit Programs*, 242
Healthy Food in Health Care Pledge,
    s52, 82, 91
    medical waste incineration, 108
    Mercury-Free Pledge, 58
    origins of, 6–7
    on waste management, 114
Health Care Without Harm sustainable
    food, 84
health determinants, ix, 239
    personal behaviors, 239
    upstream and downstream, 238–241
Health Facilities Management, 75
Health and Human Services, Department
    of, 243, 244
Healthier Hospitals Initiative (HHI),
    19–20
    Balanced Menus Challenge, 100, 225
    community health orientation, 248
    environmentally preferable purchasing,
        171, 225
    EPP priority areas, 181
    food challenges, 85–86, 100, 225
    measuring environmental performance,
        224, 226
    operating room waste, 118
    organizations enrolled, 226
    partners in, 75
    Six challenges for health systems, 225
    waste reduction challenge, 116, 117,
        118, 225
health insurance industry, 36–37
Healthy Building Network, 20, 194, 195,
    196, 204
Healthy Food in Health Care Pledge, 82
    contents of pledge, 85
Healthy Food in Health Care program, 85
Healthy People 2020 agenda, 244
heavy metals, 183
Hemstreet, H. R., 41, 207
Hippocrates, 86
Hospital Corporation of America, 14
hospital design, 20, 42

building design initiative, 20, 72
chemicals in building products, 203–204
cost-effectiveness of green construction, 74–75
Fable Hospital, 68–70, 200
green building champions, 194–198
Green Healthcare Construction Guidance Statement, 198
Kaiser Permanente, 42
lifecycle approach, 196–197
regenerative systems design, 43, 209–211
smaller hospitals, 43
tools for green building, 198–200
Westside Hospital, 191–192
windows and geothermal, 46
hospitals
changing landscape, vii–x
as energy-intensive, 12, 37–38
as nonprofits, 61–62
savings from sustainable operations, 55
Hospitals for a Healthy Environment (H2E), 9
mercury elimination, 167
partnership described, 19
Howard, J., 107
Hoyde, K., 120
Huron Valley Sinai Hospital, 102–103
hurricanes, 32

Imrie, D., 91
industrial chemicals, 132
See also green chemistry; toxic chemicals
biomagnification, 137
cleaning products, 147, 157–158
common products containing, 134
guiding principles, 143–144
hazardous and toxic, 137, 205
in health care, 134–136
impacts unstudied, 10, 136
national policy, 153–157
opposing or synergistic effects, 137
organizational chemicals policy, 144
present in humans, 11, 135, 138
product purchasing policy, 144–148
resistance by trade groups, 206–207
Toxic Substances Control Act, 10–11, 133

infants and chemical risks, 137–139
Ingram, B. L., 32
Inova Health System, 109
Institute for Healthcare Improvement, 56
insurance industry
and climate change, 36–37
Intergovernmental Panel on Climate Change (IPCC), 25
IRS rules for non-profits, 241–242, 245
ISO 14001 standard, 217–218
IT (information technology)
controlling waste, 181–182
purchasing strategies for greener electronics, 184–189
IV bags and tubing, 3–4, 141

janitorial supplies, 147, 157–158
Jevons paradox, 41
Johns Hopkins University Hospital, 117, 121
Johnson & Johnson, 231, 233

Kaiser, H., xi
Kaiser Permanente
areas prioritized for action, 22–23
chemicals priorities, 180
cleaning products, 147
climate position, 37, 38–40
Community Benefit department, 237–238
Community Health Initiatives (CHI), 249–251
computer purchasing and data center efficiency, 49–50
Denver B-cycle program, 250–251
"distributed accountability" approach, 57
early environmental awareness, xi
"Eco-Toolkit," 71, 199
energy and natural resources priorities, 180
energy use costs, 220
environmentally preferable purchasing, 56, 172–176, 178–179
Environmental Stewardship Council, xii, 57, 175, 180
environmental stewardship strategies, 5, 56, 62–63, 236–237
EPEAT standards, 187–188

Kaiser Permanente (*Cont.*)
  flame retardants on medical furniture,
    159
  food criteria, 84, 91–92, 95–96, 180
  green building design, 197
  Green Guide for Health Care, 72
  green teams, 16, 17
  hospital design, 42, 197, 210–211
  Keep IT Green teams, 50
  KP Health Connect, 51
  LEE for New Construction Gold, 207
  medical waste policy, 13, 122, 123,
    128–129
  mission and margin considerations, 62
  National Product Council, 173–174
  non-PVC construction materials,
    200–201
  Oakland hospital, 78
  paper use reduction, 164–165, 172
  parking lots, 215
  Position Statement on Green Buldings,
    199
  procurement cost myths, 67–68
  purchasing annually, 165
  PVC concerns, 2
  Rachel Carson's impact, 15–16
  recycling construction debris, 126
  recycling electronic equipment, 125
  renewable energy, 41
  response to climate change, 38–40
  safer chemicals statement, 142–143
  San Francisco Medical Center, 1, 3
  seismic-replacement hospitals, 193–194,
    199
  small hospital design, 210–211
  sourcing and standards teams (SSTs),
    174
  sustainable energy policy, 38–40
  sustainable food criteria, 84, 96–97
  Sustainable Scorecard, 169, 176
  "Targeted Ten" list of hazardous prod-
    ucts, 146–147
  tools for calculating GHG emissions, 38
  "total health" ethos, 56, 62–63
  TSCA reform, 155
  virtual office visits, 51
  Westside Hospital, 42, 191–192
Kaiser Permanente HealthConnect, 129
Kats, G., 74
King, D., 218
Kiowa County Memorial Hospital, 207
Knickman, J. R., 65
Kouletsis, J., 68, 197

landfill gas
  as energy source, 48–49
  methane emissions from, 113, 211
latex gloves, 146
Lautenberg, F., 136, 156
Leadership in Energy and Environmental
  Design (LEED), 20
  Gold-certified hospital, 191, 208, 212
Leciejewski, M. E., 80
LEED-accredited design engineers, 197
LEED for Healthcare, 73, 206–208
LEED for New Construction rating
  system, 71, 202
LEED Version 4 (v4), 206
Legacy Good Samaritan Hospital, 18
Lent, T., 198, 203, 204, 205
life cycle assessment (LCA), 223
lighting
  dimmed nighttime, 48
  light bulb upgrades, 40, 47
  patient-centered, 47–48
Lipsey, S., 33
LiveWell Colorado, 249
Lochner, V., 178–179
Luber, G., 36
Lundgren, G., 136

Makary, M. A., 117
manure digester, 46
Maring, P., 78–79, 99
Massachusetts General Hospital, 34, 210
Mayo Clinic, 120
Mazzetti Nash Lipsey Burch, 33, 43, 210
McCally, M., 135
McGinnis, J. M., 65, 239
McKinlay, J., 241

measurement of environmental
    interventions, 215–216
  audiences for reports, 228–230
  effective reporting of data, 228–230
  enterprise sustainability management
    software (ESMS), 226–228
  getting started, 216–217
  Global Reporting Initiative (GRI), 230–232
  SMART targets in priority areas, 217
  tools for, 217–224
  verification of results, 232–234
MedAssets, 169, 173
medical waste
  4Rs, 108–109
  blue wrap recycling, 120, 126–127
  community health and, 16
  electronic device recycling and reuse,
    124–125
  excess supplies to developing world, 124
  generated by hospitals, 13
  health and environmental consequences
    of, 112–114
  incineration. See medical waste
    incinerators
  Kaiser Permanente best practices,
    128–129
  major hospital waste streams, 116–118
  mixing noninfectious wastes with,
    13–14, 57, 118, 119, 126
  operating room waste, 117–120
  per staffed bed per day, 107
  recycling abroad, 124
  reformulating operating room packs,
    118–120
  reprocessing single-use devices, 120–123
  reusable sharps containers, 123, 128
  reusable surgical textiles, 122
  segregation of waste streams, 109–112
  single-use device (SUD) recycling,
    120–123
  source reduction, 114–115
  successes, 14
  "syringe tide," 16
  types of, 108, 109, 110–111
  "waste audits," 106

  waste management as key, 107
  waste management plan, 114–116
  Waste Minimization Team, 57
  waste stream analysis, 115
medical waste incinerators, 5, 108
  decreases recently, 114
  dioxin pollution from, 6
  disposal issues, 13
  in existence, 10
  toxins released, 113
Medicare/Medicaid reimbursement issues, 73
MedShare, 124, 125–126
MedWish, 124
mercury, 10
  atmospheric impact, 57
  costs of cleanups after spills, 57–58
  environmentally preferable purchasing,
    167
  policies eliminating, 22, 57
  "total cost of ownership," 57–58
Messervy, J., 33, 34, 210
methane emissions, 27, 28, 28, 113
Metro West Medical Center (Framingham,
    MA), 100–101, 126–127
Michigan Health and Hospitals
    Association, 98
Michigan's Metro Health Hospital, 122
Midmark, 159
Mount Sinai School of Medicine, 11
MRSA (methicillin-resistant staph
    aureus), 90

National Health Service (United
    Kingdom), 221–222, 222
National Healthy Food Financing
    Initiative, 248
National Prevention Strategy, 243–244
National Prevention and Wellness Trust, 248
National Report on Human Exposure to
    Environmental Chemicals, 11
National Research Council (NRC), 137
National Resource Defense Council, 183
National Strategy for Quality
    Improvement in Health Care, 243
natural resources, 60

Navigant Research, 150
neonatal intensive care units (NICUs), 1–4
Newman, T., 90
New York-Presbyterian Healthcare system, 109
New York University's Langone Hospital, 32
nonprofit health care, 61–62
Novation, 143

Obama, Michelle, 96, 248
obesity epidemic, 80–81
    early exposure to endocrine-disrupting chemicals, 139
    Michigan example, 98
    upstream and downstream factors, 241
operating room waste management, 117–118
    reformulating operating room packs, 118–120
    St. Vincent Medical Center, 127
Oregon Health and Science University, 101, 207
Orndoff, D., 207, 208
overweight and obesity, 86–87

paper use reduction
    federal government, 166
    Kaiser Permanente, 164–165, 172
    recycled-content (RC) copy paper, 172
parking garages, 42
Partners HealthCare, 33–34, 210
Partnership for a Healthier America, 96, 248
Patton, S., xii
Pearl, R., 63–64
Pencheon, D., 221–222
perfluorochemicals, 135, 138
Perkins + Will, 43, 194, 205, 210
Pesticides in the Diets of Infants and Children, 137
Peters, B., 98
pharmaceuticals
    carbon-intensive nature, 221–222
pharmaceutical waste, 110
Pharos Project, 204–205
Physicians for Social Responsibility (PSR), 90, 135, 142

Pollution Prevention Act, 148
poop-power project, 46
poor health, main causes of, ix
Portfolio Manager, 38, 218–219
    greenhouse gas emissions, 220
Pott, P., 132
Practice Greenhealth
    Energy Impact Calculator, 220
    Environmental Leadership Circle, 126
    goals, 9
    Greening the OR Initiative, 118, 119
    Greening the Supply Chain initiative, 168
    greenwashing advice, 185
    harmful chemicals, 142
    origins, 8, 19
    standardized list of environmental questions, 169, 170
    supplier questionnaire, 168–169, 170, 179
    Sustainability Benchmark Report, 22, 228
    sustainable food scorecard, 97
    tools for measuring GHGs, 38
    waste management awards, 122
Precautionary Principle, 142
    in purchasing policy, 175
premature death, causes of, 239
Premier, Inc., 143, 188
President's Cancer Panel, 88, 136
    on TSCA, 155
Press, S., 50
Prestbo, J., 61
prevention paradigm, 64–67
Prevention and Public Health Fund, 243
procurement
    cost myths, 67–68
product purchasing policy, 144–148
    supplier disclosure scorecard, 145, 179
Program on Reproductive Health and the Environment, 88
Providence Health and Services, 108
public health policy, 242–245
Public Library of Materials (PLUM), 151
Puget Sound Food Network, 98
purchasing policy, 71–72

for chemical and hazardous products,
    144–148
Environmental Product Declarations
    (EPDs), 223–224
group purchasing organizations
    (GPOs), 167–168
health care supplies annual cost, 165
paper use reduction, 164–165
standardized environment questions, 170
Puyallup Medical Center, 73, 207, 212–213
PVC (polyvinyl chloride) plastics, 2
elimination from hospital building
    materials, 200–201
incineration, 6, 114
Kaiser Permanente approach, 57, 141
reduction policies, 22
substitutes for, 6
switching to PVC-free, 18
ubiquitous nature in health care, 6, 204

Rady Children's Hospital, 56
RCRA hazardous waste, 110
recycling
electronic products, dangers of, 183
recycling programs, 22
blue wrap, 120, 126–127
construction debris, 125–126
to developing world, 124
electronic devices, 124–125
Kaiser Permanente best practices, 128–129
potential for, 107
recyclables defined, 111
single-use devices (SUDs), 120–123
St. Vincent Medical Center, 127
Redemtech (now Arrow Value Recovery), 125
regenerative systems design, 43, 209–211
Regional Produce Purchasing Project, 99
regulated medical waste (RMW) stream,
    109
measures for segregating, 112
operating room waste, 119
RMW defined, 110
renewable energy, 41
Gundersen, 45–46
renewable energy certificates (RECs), 41

Resource Conservation and Recovery Act
    (1976), 166
retrocommissioning audits, 44–45
Rich, J., 44, 45, 46–47
Ridgeview Medical Center, 158
Rose, J., 42

Sadler, B. L., 56
Safe Chemicals Act, 156
Safer Chemicals Healthy Families
    coalition, 156
San Francisco VA Hospital, 101
Savitz, A., 59
Schettler, Ted, 2–3, 81
School of Nursing at University of Texas at
    Houston, 18–19
Science and Environmental Health
    Network, 3, 81
Scientific Certification Systems, 186
Seattle Children's Hospital, 50–51
seismic safety goals, 193–194
Setting Healthcare's Environmental
    Agenda conference, 70–72, 195–196
Silent Spring (Carson), 15, 87
single-use device (SUD) recycling, 120–123
social capital, 60
solar energy, 41
solid oxide fuel cells, 41
Solomon, L., 63, 248
source reduction, 114–115
sourcing and standards teams (SSTs), 174
Spaulding Rehabilitation Hospital, 33–34,
    210
St. Elizabeth's Medical Center, 102
Stericycle, 114
Stewart, J., xi–xii
Stockholm Convention on Persistent
    Organic Pollutants, 154
St. Vincent Medical Center, 127
sugar-sweetened beverages (SSBs), 101–103
sustainability
in building design, 196, 208–209
in food production, 84
goals and early efforts, 14–20
Sustainability Benchmark Report, 22, 228

sustainability performance, 61
Sustainability Roadmap for Hospitals
    project, 115
Sustainability Scorecard, 169, 176, 188
sustainable chemistry. *See* green chemistry
Sustainable Fabrics Alliance, 159
Sustainable Food Scorecard, 96–97
Sutton, P., 88
Sweden, 218

Tellus Institute, 230
Tenet Healthcare, 231–232
Thompson, J., 44, 47
Thompson, T. J., 97
total health concept, xi, 56, 62, *63*, 237
toxic chemicals, 10–11
    See also industrial chemicals
    author tested for, 11
    California Proposition65, 152
    chemical agents in hospitals, 13
    Green Guide for Health Care listings,
        203–204
    impact of, 11
    lack of health care sector expertise on,
        141–142
    resistance by trade groups, 206–207
Toxic Substances Control Act (TSCA),
    10–11, 133, 147
    analyzed, 153–157
    reform of, 155–157
Toxics Use Reduction Institute, 144
transportation
    community health, 248
    costs, 50–51
    Denver B-cycle program, 250–251
triple bottom line, 58–61, 196–197
Trust for America's Health, 36
Tyson, B. J., xi

Ulrich, R., 208
UN Environment Program, 230
UN Food and Agriculture Organization
    (FAO), 93
UN Global Compact, 232

Union Carbide Bhopal disaster, 5
universal coverage, 66
universal waste, 111
University of California, San Francisco
    (UCSF) Medical Center, 90, 101
University of Minnesota Medical Center
    (UMMC), Fairview, 119–120, 122
US Department of Agriculture (USDA),
    186
US Green Building Council
    third-party verified EPDs, 224
US Green Building Council (USGBC), 20,
    71, 202, 206
utility bill payment systems, 218
    GHG inventory based on, 221

vehicle emissions, 40
    health care trips, 221
Vickers, S., 18, 231
Villarante, J., 90–91
vinyl flooring, 194–195
Vittori, G., 71, 72, 195–197, 198, 203

Walsh, Bill, 195, 204
Warner, J. C., 148
waste management plan, 114–116
    See also medical waste
    ten steps, 115–116
water use, 13
    bottled water use, 52
    Kaiser Permanente priorities, 180
    Portfolio Manager for tracking, 219
West Nile virus, 35
Westside Medical Center (Hillsboro,
    Oregon), 42, 191–192, 208
Whittaker, P., 158
WHO Commission on Social
    Determinants of Health, 239
Wilkening, T., 158
Williams, H., 200–201
Williams-Russo, P., 65
Wilson, M., 151
World Health Organization (WHO), 12,
    35, 134

Made in the USA
Las Vegas, NV
05 May 2023

71522449R00155